THE CRISIS
IN DRUG
PROHIBITION

THE CRISIS IN DRUG PROHIBITION

EDITED BY DAVID BOAZ

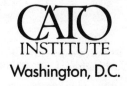

INSTITUTE

Washington, D.C.

Library of Congress Cataloging-in-Publication Data

The Crisis in drug prohibition / edited by David Boaz.
    p. cm.
    Includes bibliographical references and index.
    ISBN 0-932790-77-1
    1. Narcotics, Control of—United States. 2. Narcotic laws—United
States. 3. Decriminalization—United States. I. Boaz, David, 1953—
HV5825.C76   1990
363.4′5′0973— dc20   90-2128
                                                   CIP

Printed in the United States of America.

CATO INSTITUTE
224 Second Street, S.E.
Washington, D.C. 20003

Contents

Preface

In June 1989 the Cato Institute sponsored a Washington forum at which four leading critics of drug prohibition presented their views: David Boaz, executive vice president of the Cato Institute; Ethan A. Nadelmann, professor of politics at Princeton University; James Ostrowski, author of a Cato study on prohibition; and Kurt Schmoke, mayor of Baltimore.

Since that time the drug war has expanded in a number of ways. More money is being spent on drug prohibition at the federal, state, and local level. More drugs are being interdicted at our borders, even as more drugs cross those borders. More drug dealers, more policemen, and more bystanders are being killed in black-market violence. And the U.S. military, searching for a rationale for its $300 billion budget in the post–Cold War era, is increasingly enthusiastic about enlisting in the drug war.

At the same time, it has become increasingly obvious that the drug war is unwinnable, and more and more Americans have concluded that some sort of alternative to prohibition is needed. Former secretary of state George Shultz and federal judge Robert Sweet have joined an impressive group of conscientious objectors: Nobel laureate Milton Friedman, economists Thomas Sowell and Gary Becker, journalists Anthony Lewis, William F. Buckley, Jr., Richard Cohen, Stephen Chapman, and Mike Royko, physicians Kildare Clarke and Nancy Lord, elected officials Joseph Galiber and Bill Mathesius, and drug policy researchers Arnold Trebach and Stephen Wisotsky, to name only a few. According to polls in early 1990, they were joined by some 30 percent of the American people, up from 10 percent just 18 months earlier.

Although more and more people are coming to understand the counterproductive effects of drug prohibition, there are significant differences among the proposed alternatives. Many, however, are converging on the idea that decriminalization or legalization of the use and sale of drugs would solve most of what we loosely call "the drug problem": crime, corruption, AIDS, and the destruction of inner-city communities.

As the costs of drug prohibition become more apparent, the Cato Institute is pleased to present this collection of essays by distinguished critics. We hope that it will lead to further debate about alternatives to prohibition.

EDWARD H. CRANE
President
Cato Institute

The Consequences of Prohibition

David Boaz

The Army is training young surgeons to handle battlefield wounds by sending them to the emergency room at a Los Angeles ghetto hospital inundated with victims of gang violence—where they will find large numbers of wounds caused by high-velocity automatic and semiautomatic gunfire.

Colombia is in a state of civil war, and hundreds of civilians died in the American attempt to bring accused drug dealer Manuel Noriega to trial.

In Washington, D.C., a reading teacher, trying to persuade her fourth-graders to read at home, urges them to take a pillow and read in the bathtub—the last place a stray bullet from the drug wars would be likely to reach.

And some people still say that *ending* drug prohibition would be a dangerous social experiment!

This essay has a very simple thesis: Alcohol didn't cause the high crime rates of the 1920s, prohibition did. And drugs don't cause today's alarming crime rates, drug prohibition does.

What are the effects of prohibition? (Drug prohibition is specifically at issue here, but the analysis applies to prohibition of almost any substance or activity.) The first result is crime. This is a very simple matter of economics. Drug laws reduce the number of suppliers and thereby the supply of drugs, driving up their price. The danger of arrest for the seller adds a risk premium to the price. The higher price means that users often commit crimes to pay for a habit that would be easily affordable if drugs were legal. Heroin, cocaine, and other substances would cost much less if they were legal. Experts estimate that at least half of the violent crime in major U.S. cities is committed by users as a result of drug prohibition.

David Boaz is executive vice president of the Cato Institute.

1

Crime also results from another factor: dealers have no nonviolent way to settle disputes with each other. We don't see shootouts in the automobile business or even in the liquor or the tobacco business. But if a drug dealer has a quarrel with another dealer, he can't sue, he can't go to court, he has no recourse except violence. It is that kind of black-market violence that has garnered most of the headlines and propelled Washington's murder rate to two consecutive annual records since the federal government decided to make Washington a model of drug enforcement.

The second effect of prohibition is corruption. Prohibition raises prices, which leads to extraordinary profits, which are an irresistible temptation to policemen, customs officers, Latin American officials, and others. We should be shocked not that there are Miami policemen on the take but that there are some Miami policemen not on the take. Policemen make $35,000 a year and have to arrest people who are driving cars worth several times that. Should we be surprised that some of the drug money trickles down into the pockets of policemen?

The third result, and one that is often underestimated, is bringing buyers into contact with criminals. The very illegality of the drug business attracts people who are already criminals. As conservatives say about guns, if drugs are outlawed, only outlaws will sell drugs. The decent people who would like to sell drugs the way they might sell liquor are squeezed out of an increasingly violent business. If you buy alcohol, you don't have to deal with criminals.

If a student buys marijuana on a college campus, he may not have to deal with criminals, but the person he buys it from probably does deal with criminals. And if a high school student buys drugs, there is a very good chance that the people he's buying them from—the people who are bringing drugs right to his doorstep, to his housing project, to his schoolyard—are hardened criminals who have gone into the drug business precisely because it is illegal. One of the strongest arguments for legalization is to divorce drug use from involvement in a criminal culture.

The criminal culture associated with drugs has resulted in the destruction of many inner-city communities. Uneducated young people in inner cities face three choices: welfare, low-wage work, or drug dealing, which, as public officials and the media constantly remind us, can pay thousands of dollars a week. Is it any wonder

2

that young people with entrepreneurial skills enter the drug business? When criminals are the most successful people in a community, the effect on that community's natural order is devastating. The authority of parents, schools, religious leaders, and (legal) businesspeople is undermined, and violent criminals become role models.

The fourth effect is the creation of stronger drugs. Writing in *National Review*, Richard Cowan has promulgated what he calls the iron law of prohibition: The more intense the law enforcement, the more potent the drugs. If a dealer can smuggle only one suitcase full of drugs into the United States or drive only one car full of drugs into Baltimore, which would he rather be carrying—marijuana, coca leaves, cocaine, or crack? He gets more dollars for the bulk if he carries more potent drugs. The same thing happened during Prohibition; the production of beer declined while spirits accounted for a larger part of total alcohol consumption.

When one advocates drug legalization, a standard question is, "Well, marijuana is one thing, maybe even cocaine, but are you seriously saying you would legalize crack?" The answer is that crack is almost entirely a product of prohibition. It probably would not exist if drugs had been legal for the past 20 years.

The fifth result of drug prohibition is the spread of AIDS. About 25 percent of AIDS cases are contracted through intravenous drug use—but it isn't the chemicals in the drugs that cause AIDS, it's the sharing of needles. Needles are shared because they're illegal and difficult to obtain. In Hong Kong, where needles are available in drugstores, as of 1987 there were no cases of AIDS among drug users.

The sixth effect of prohibition is abuses of civil liberties. We have heard a lot recently about Zero Tolerance and the seizure of cars and boats because a small amount of marijuana or cocaine was allegedly found. I recall a time in this country when the government was allowed to punish people only after they had been convicted in a court of law. It now appears that the drug authorities can punish American citizens by seizing their cars or boats, not after indictment—much less conviction—but after nothing more than an allegation by a police officer. Whatever happened to the presumption of innocence?

We have seen several dramatic examples of civil liberties abuses in the drug war recently. A woman in Rochester, New York, had

3

her house seized by U.S. marshals because her son had allegedly sold marijuana in the house without her knowledge. She couldn't make bail for her son because she no longer owned the house she would have used for collateral. In Detroit, authorities seized more than $4,000 from a grocery cash register after finding traces of cocaine on three $1 bills—a practice that ought to strike fear into the heart of every urban retailer.

There is an inherent problem of civil liberties abuses in victimless crimes, as Randy Barnett noted in the Pacific Research Institute book *Dealing with Drugs*. In most crimes, such as robbery or rape, there is a person who in our legal system is called the complaining witness: the person who was robbed or raped and complains to the police that a crime has been committed. In a drug purchase, neither party to the transaction complains. Now what does that mean? It means there are no witnesses who complain about the problem so the police have to get their evidence some other way. Policemen have to start going undercover, and that leads to entrapment, wire-tapping, and all sorts of things that border on civil liberties abuses—and usually end up crossing the border.

The seventh result of prohibition is a feeling of futility. The drug war simply isn't working. The *Washington Post* reported recently:

> Faced with a growing epidemic of violence in the past year, District officials have committed more money and man-power than ever before to stemming the flow of drugs in the city.
> Police officers in six of the city's seven districts were ordered to work six days a week. Officers who had been assigned to desk jobs for the past 10 years were required to do part-time patrol duty. And 50 officers were assigned to a new narcotics unit east of the Anacostia River, an area hit especially hard by drug violence.

They also arrested and convicted the biggest cocaine dealer in town and all his colleagues. And what were the results? "The drug's price has remained stable, its potency high and its supply plentiful."

The story is the same across the country. Every year federal agents interdict more drugs entering the country than ever before. Every month the biggest drug bust in history is announced. And drugs continue to be available on Wall Street, in Harlem, and in rural Iowa.

4

Some say that much of today's support for legalization is merely a sign of frustration. Well, frustration is a rational response to futility. It's quite understandable that people have become frustrated with the continuing failure of new enforcement policies.

A government involved in a war it isn't winning has two basic choices—escalate or get out—and we're seeing a lot of proposals for escalation.

Former New York mayor Ed Koch has proposed strip searching every person entering the United States from South America or Southeast Asia. Members of the D.C. City Council have called for the National Guard to occupy the capital city of the United States. Congress has bravely called for the death penalty for drug sellers.

Jesse Jackson wants to bring the troops home from Europe and use them to ring our southern border. The police chief of Los Angeles wants to invade Colombia.

President Reagan's White House drug adviser and the *Wall Street Journal* editorial page have called for arresting small-time users. The *Journal*, with its usual spirit, urged the government to "crush the users"; that's 23 million Americans. The Justice Department wants to double our prison capacity even though we already have far more people in prison as a percentage of our population than any other industrialized country except South Africa. Former attorney general Edwin Meese III and others want to drug test all workers.

The Customs Service asked for authorization to "use appropriate force" to compel planes suspected of carrying drugs to land. Former commissioner William von Raab clarified, in case there was any doubt, that yes, he meant that if customs agents couldn't determine what a plane was up to, he wanted them to have the authority to shoot the plane down and then find out if it was carrying drugs. In 1988 that proposal was considered so ridiculous that even Ed Meese's Justice Department, not exactly a hotbed of civil libertarians, rejected it out of hand. By 1989 the idea had been approved by a majority of the U.S. Senate.

Those rather frightening ideas represent one response to the futility of the drug war.

The more sensible response, it seems to me, is to decriminalize drugs—to de-escalate the war, to realize that trying to wage war on 23 million Americans who are obviously very committed to certain recreational activities is not going to be any more successful than Prohibition was. A lot of people use drugs peacefully and safely for recreation and will not go along with Zero Tolerance. They will continue to find sources of drugs. The problems caused by prohibition are not going to be solved by stepped-up enforcement.

How exactly would we legalize drugs? Defenders of drug prohibition apparently consider that a devastating question, but it doesn't strike me as particularly difficult. Our society has had a lot of experience with legal dangerous drugs, particularly alcohol and tobacco, and we can draw on that experience when we legalize marijuana, cocaine, and heroin.

Some critics of prohibition would legalize only "soft" drugs— just marijuana in many cases. That policy would not eliminate the tremendous problems that prohibition has created. As long as drugs that people very much want remain illegal, a black market will exist. If our goal is to rid our cities of crime and corruption, it would make more sense to legalize cocaine and heroin while leaving marijuana illegal than vice versa. The lesson of alcohol prohibition in the 1920s and the prohibition of other drugs today is that prohibition creates more problems than it solves. We should legalize all recreational drugs.

Then what? When we legalize drugs, we will in all likelihood apply the alcohol model. That is, marijuana, cocaine, and heroin would be sold only in specially licensed stores—perhaps in liquor stores, perhaps in a new kind of drugstore. Warning labels would be posted in the stores and on the packages. It would be illegal to sell drugs to minors, now defined as anyone under 21. It would be illegal to advertise drugs on television and possibly even in print. Driving under the influence of drugs would be illegal, and there would be added penalties for committing other crimes under their influence, as is the case with alcohol.

It is quite possible that such a distribution system would be *less* likely to attract young people to drug use than is the current system of schoolyard pushers offering free samples. Teenagers today can get liquor if they try, and we shouldn't assume that a minimum purchasing age would keep other drugs out of their hands. But we don't see many liquor pushers peddling their wares on playgrounds. Getting the drug business out of our schoolyards and streets is an important benefit of legalization.

It is probable that drug use would initially increase. Prices would be much lower, and drugs would be more readily available to adults

6

who prefer not to break the law. But those drugs would be safer—when was the last report of a liquor store selling gin cut with formaldehyde?—and people would be able to regulate their intake more carefully.

In the long run, however, I foresee declining drug use and weaker drugs. Consider the divergent trends in legal and illegal drugs today. Illegal drugs keep getting stronger—crack, PCP, ecstasy, ice, designer drugs—as a result of the iron law of prohibition. But legal drugs are getting weaker—low-tar cigarettes, nonalcoholic beer (which contains less than 0.5 percent alcohol), wine coolers. About 41 million Americans have quit smoking, and sales of spirits are declining; beer and wine keep the alcohol industry stable. As Americans become more health conscious, they are turning away from drugs. Drug education could do more to encourage that trend if it were separated from law enforcement.

By reducing crime, drug legalization would greatly increase the safety of our neighborhoods. If would take the astronomical profits out of the drug trade, and the Colombian cartel would collapse like a punctured balloon. Drugs would be sold by Fortune 500 companies and friendly corner merchants, not by Mafiosi and 16-year-olds with BMWs and guns. Legalization would put an end to the corruption that has engulfed so many Latin American countries and tainted the Miami police and U.S. soldiers in Central America.

Finally, although I believe that health and safety considerations should lead anyone to support drug legalization, let me make a philosophical point. People have rights that governments may not violate. Thomas Jefferson defined them as the rights of life, liberty, and the pursuit of happiness. I would say that people have the right to live their lives in any way they choose as long as they don't violate the rights of others. What right could be more basic, more inherent in human nature, than the right to choose what substances to put in one's own body? Whether we're talking about alcohol, tobacco, laetrile, AZT, saturated fat, or cocaine, that is a decision that should be made by the individual, not the government. If government can tell us what we can put into our own bodies, what can it not tell us? What limits on government action are there?

Legalization would not solve all of America's drug problems, but it would make our cities safer, make drug use healthier, eliminate a major source of revenue for organized crime, reduce corruption here and abroad, and make honest work more attractive to inner-city youth—pretty good results for any reform.

Drugs: A Problem of Health and Economics

Kurt L. Schmoke

Has the time come to add America's "war on drugs" to the long list of history's follies? In the view of historian Barbara Tuchman, to qualify as folly, a policy must not only be unsuccessful, it must be plainly against the interests of those in whose name it is being carried out. And folly has one more characteristic: Nobody wants to recognize it.

Whether the drug policies of the United States have reached the point of folly, I'm not prepared to say. But this much seems apparent: Political maturity, intellectual honesty and justifiable concern about drug-related violence make raising the question long overdue.

This is why I asked the U.S. Conference of Mayors last month to adopt a resolution calling upon Congress to hold hearings on whether to decriminalize narcotics.

The details—which drugs would be legalized, and how and by whom they could be purchased—would be left to Congress and state legislatures to decide after first concluding on the basis of research and testimony that some form of decriminalization is warranted.

Many who oppose decriminalization argue that it will serve as an open invitation to use drugs. If there is evidence to that effect, then it should be dispassionately presented to Congress and other policymakers, but it should not stand in the way of a public debate about decriminalization.

The time has come to admit that the emperor has no clothes. The war on drugs is being lost, notwithstanding President Reagan's recent claim that we are digging our way out. And continuing our

Kurt L. Schmoke is mayor of Baltimore.
This article is reprinted, with permission, from the *Washington Post*, May 15, 1988.

9

present policy—even with more money—is unlikely to make any difference.

There are three basic arguments in favor of decriminalization: libertarianism, economics and health. I don't subscribe to the libertarian view that people should have a right to injure themselves with drugs if they so choose. Drugs—even if decriminalized—also pose a danger to third parties. But the other two arguments are compelling enough for Congress at least to study the question.

Economics

Just as Prohibition banned something millions of people want, our current drug laws make it illegal to possess a commodity that is in very high demand. As a result, the price of that commodity has soared far beyond its true cost.

This has led to enormous profits from illegal drugs and turned drug trafficking into the criminal enterprise of choice for pushers and manufacturers alike.

I know this because for more than seven years I made a living putting people in jail. As an assistant U.S. attorney, and later state's attorney for Baltimore, I prosecuted and won convictions against thousands of defendants for drug-related crimes. Those crimes included murder of police officers and civilians; the victims included innocent bystanders and children caught up in criminal enterprises whose danger they could never appreciate.

During my years as a prosecutor, as I watched drug crime change the character of America's cities, I learned some important lessons. First, drug traffickers—no matter how high-up or how venal— care very little about the sanctions of the criminal-justice system. Going to jail is just part of the cost of doing business. It's a nuisance, not a deterrent.

Second, drug dealers fear one another far more than they fear law-enforcement officials. They know that the police must give them due process, but competing drug dealers will kill them at a moment's notice.

Finally, profit is the engine driving drug trafficking. Neither criminal sanctions nor even the competitive business practices (murder, extortion, kidnapping) of their fellow dealers have much, if any, effect on people who trade in drugs.

But take the profit out of their enterprise—and you'll get their attention. Perhaps it's time to fight the crime epidemic associated

10

with drug trafficking by communicating with the drug under-ground in the only language they understand: Money.

Decriminalization would take the profit out of drugs and greatly reduce, if not eliminate, the drug-related violence that is currently plaguing our streets. Decriminalization will not solve this country's drug abuse problem, but it could solve our most intractable crime problem.

It is very easy for people living in communities where drugs are not a problem (and those are becoming fewer all the time) to argue that drug-related violence cannot justify decriminalization. But if you have to live with that violence day in and day out—as millions of people in large urban areas do—and live in terror of being gunned down, robbed or assaulted, or having the same occur to one of your loved ones, you soon start wanting results.

Taking the profit out of drugs would have a detrimental impact on those who are now producing and selling drugs. Drug lords would no longer risk prison for a commodity that was not making them a profit.

Health

Some will argue that the public-health risks from drugs will only worsen if they are decriminalized. Again, this is a question Congress would need to resolve, but there is every reason to believe that decriminalization would improve public health.

First, violent crime associated with illegal sale of drugs would fall dramatically. For those who doubt that, imagine how violent crime would increase if we once again made the use and sale of alcohol illegal.

Second, decriminalization would allow billions of dollars now used for interdiction and enforcement to be redirected toward prevention and treatment.

Smoking kills over 300,000 people every year, but we have made the policy decision to treat tobacco as a health problem, not a crime problem, and we are making real progress. The number of people smoking continues to fall because of a concerted public education campaign about the health effects of smoking.

There is no reason that we could not do the same with drugs. And then we could find the money we need to educate our young people on the harmful effects of drugs and treat those who are currently addicted, instead of engaging in a wildly expensive cat-and-mouse game that the mouse is winning 90 percent of the time.

To make matters worse, the Reagan administration has continuously tried to cut drug programs aimed at the prevention and treatment of drug abuse. It was Congress, through its passage of the Anti-Drug Abuse Act of 1986, that enabled the United States to make an even modestly credible effort to treat and prevent drug abuse. But it is doubtful that even the effort of Congress will make much difference. Several hundred million dollars to fight the health effects of an enterprise earning billions is not sufficient. Only by applying a substantial portion of the more than three billion dollars invested in the total federal drug program can we begin to treat those currently addicted—many of whom now have AIDS—and properly educate our children about the harmful effects of drugs.

Many political and opinion leaders will resist the notion that our current drug policy is folly, and perhaps they're right. But all the signs are there: We're spending billions of dollars in an effort that is enriching the very people we're trying to stop. And in the meantime, millions of people continue to use drugs and millions more have lost all confidence that they can live securely in their neighborhoods.

It takes great maturity and willpower for a society to step back from a policy that on the surface seems noble and justified, but in reality has only compounded the problem it is attempting to solve. On the subject of drugs, such maturity and willpower may now be in order. At the very least, we need a sober national debate on the subject.

The Case for Legalization

Ethan A. Nadelmann

What can be done about the "drug problem"? Despite frequent proclamations of war and dramatic increases in government funding and resources in recent years, there are many indications that the problem is not going away and may even be growing worse. During the past year alone, more than thirty million Americans violated the drug laws on literally billions of occasions. Drug-treatment programs in many cities are turning people away for lack of space and funding. In Washington, D.C., drug-related killings, largely of one drug dealer by another, are held responsible for a doubling in the homicide rate over the past year. In New York and elsewhere, courts and prisons are clogged with a virtually limitless supply of drug-law violators. In large cities and small towns alike, corruption of policemen and other criminal-justice officials by drug traffickers is rampant.

President Reagan and the First Lady are not alone in supporting increasingly repressive and expensive anti-drug measures and in believing that the war against drugs can be won. Indeed, no "war" proclaimed by an American leader during the past forty years has garnered such sweeping bipartisan support; on this issue, liberals and conservatives are often indistinguishable. The fiercest disputes are not over objectives or even broad strategies but over turf and tactics. Democratic politicians push for the appointment of a "drug czar" to oversee all drug policy and blame the Administration for not applying sufficient pressure and sanctions against the foreign drug-producing countries. Republicans try to gain the upper hand by daring Democrats to support more widespread drug testing, increasingly powerful law-enforcement measures, and the death

Ethan A. Nadelmann is assistant professor of politics and public affairs at the Woodrow Wilson School of Public and International Affairs at Princeton University.
This article is reprinted, with permission, from the Summer 1988 issue of the *Public Interest*.

penalty for various drug-related offenses. But on the more fundamental issues of what this war is about, and what strategies are most likely to prove successful in the long run, no real debate—much less vocal dissent—can be heard.

If there were a serious public debate on this issue, far more attention would be given to one policy option that has just begun to be seriously considered but that may well prove more successful than anything currently being implemented or proposed: legalization. Politicians and public officials remain hesitant even to mention the word, except to dismiss it contemptuously as a capitulation to the drug traffickers. Most Americans perceive drug legalization as an invitation to drug-infested anarchy. Even the civil-liberties groups shy away from this issue, limiting their input primarily to the drug-testing debate. The minority communities in the ghetto, for whom repealing the drug laws would promise the greatest benefits, fail to recognize the costs of our drug-prohibition policies. And the typical middle-class American, who hopes only that his children will not succumb to drug abuse, tends to favor any measures that he believes will make illegal drugs less accessible to them. Yet when one seriously compares the advantages and disadvantages of the legalization strategy with those of current and planned policies, abundant evidence suggests that legalization may well be the optimal strategy for tackling the drug problem.

Interestingly, public support for repealing the drug-prohibition laws has traditionally come primarily from the conservative end of the political spectrum: Milton Friedman, Ernest van den Haag, William F. Buckley, and the editors of the *Economist* have all supported it. Less vocal support comes from many liberals, politicians not among them, who are disturbed by the infringements on individual liberty posed by the drug laws. There is also a significant silent constituency in favor of repeal, found especially among criminal-justice officials, intelligence analysts, military interdictors, and criminal-justice scholars who have spent a considerable amount of time thinking about the problem. More often than not, however, job-security considerations, combined with an awareness that they can do little to change official policies, ensure that their views remain discreet and off the record.

During the spring of 1988, however, legalization suddenly began to be seriously considered as a policy option; the pros and cons of legalization were discussed on the front pages of leading newspapers and news magazines and were debated on national television programs. Although the argument for legalization was not new, two factors seem to have been primarily responsible for the blitz of media coverage: an intellectual rationale for legalization—the first provided in decades—appeared in my article in the Spring issue of *Foreign Policy* magazine; more important, political legitimacy was subsequently bestowed upon the legalization option when Baltimore Mayor Kurt Schmoke, speaking to the National Conference of Mayors, noted the potential benefits of drug legalization and asked that the merits of legalization be debated in congressional hearings.

The idea of legalizing drugs was quickly denounced by most politicians across the political spectrum; nevertheless, the case for legalization appealed to many Americans. The prominent media coverage lent an aura of respectability to arguments that just a month earlier had seemed to be beyond the political pale. Despite the tendency of many journalists to caricature the legalization argument, at long last the issue had been joined. Various politicians, law-enforcement officials, health experts, and scholars came out in favor of drug legalization—or at least wanted to debate the matter seriously. On Capitol Hill, three or four congressmen seconded the call for a debate. According to some congressional staffers, two dozen additional legislators would have wanted to debate the issue, had the question arisen after rather than before the upcoming elections. Unable to oppose a mere hearing on the issue, Congressman Charles Rangel, chairman of the House Select Committee on Narcotics Abuse and Control, declared his willingness to convene his committee in Baltimore to consider the legalization option.

There is, of course, no single legalization strategy. At one extreme is the libertarian vision of virtually no government restraints on the production and sale of drugs or any psychoactive substances, except perhaps around the fringes, such as prohibiting sales to children. At the other extreme is total government control over the production and sale of these goods. In between lies a strategy that may prove more successful than anything yet tried in stemming the problems of drug abuse and drug-related violence, corruption, sickness, and suffering. It is one in which government makes most of the substances that are now banned legally available to competent adults, exercises strong regulatory powers over all large-scale

15

production and sale of drugs, makes drug-treatment programs available to all who need them, and offers honest drug-education programs to children. This strategy, it is worth noting, would also result in a net benefit to public treasuries of at least ten billion dollars a year, and perhaps much more.

There are three reasons why it is important to think about legalization scenarios, even though most Americans remain hostile to the idea. First, current drug-control policies have failed, are failing, and will continue to fail, in good part because they are fundamentally flawed. Second, many drug-control efforts are not only failing but also proving highly costly and counterproductive; indeed, many of the drug-related evils that Americans identify as part and parcel of the "drug problem" are in fact caused by our drug-prohibition policies. Third, there is good reason to believe that repealing many of the drug laws would not lead, as many people fear, to a dramatic rise in drug abuse. In this essay I expand on each of these reasons for considering the legalization option. Government efforts to deal with the drug problem will succeed only if the rhetoric and crusading mentality that now dominate drug policy are replaced by reasoned and logical analysis.

Why Current Drug Policies Fail

Most proposals for dealing with the drug problem today reflect a desire to point the finger at those most removed from one's home and area of expertise. New York Mayor Ed Koch, Florida Congressman Larry Smith, and Harlem Congressman Charles Rangel, who recognize government's inability to deal with the drug problem in the cities, are among the most vocal supporters of punishing foreign drug-producing countries and stepping up interdiction efforts. Foreign leaders and U.S. State Department and drug-enforcement officials stationed abroad, on the other hand, who understand all too well why it is impossible to crack down successfully on illicit drug production outside the United States, are the most vigorous advocates of domestic enforcement and demand-reduction efforts within the United States. In between, those agencies charged with drug interdiction, from the Coast Guard and U.S. Customs Service to the U.S. military, know that they will never succeed in capturing more than a small percentage of the illicit drugs being smuggled into the United States. Not surprisingly, they point their fingers in both directions. The solution, they promise, lies in greater source-control efforts abroad and greater demand-reduction efforts at home.

Trying to pass the buck is always understandable. But in each of these cases, the officials are half right and half wrong—half right in recognizing that they can do little to affect their end of the drug problem, given the suppositions and constraints of current drug-control strategies; half wrong (if we assume that their finger pointing is sincere) in expecting that the solution lies elsewhere. It would be wrong, however, to assume that the public posturing of many officials reflects their real views. Many of them privately acknowledge the futility of all current drug-control strategies and wonder whether radically different options, such as legalization, might not prove more successful in dealing with the drug problem. The political climate pervading this issue is such, however, that merely to ask that alternatives to current policies be considered is to incur a great political risk.

By most accounts, the dramatic increase in drug-enforcement efforts over the past few years has had little effect on the illicit drug market in the United States. The mere existence of drug-prohibition laws, combined with a minimal level of law-enforcement resources, is sufficient to maintain the price of illicit drugs at a level significantly higher than it would be if there were no such laws. Drug laws and enforcement also reduce the availability of illicit drugs, most notably in parts of the United States where demand is relatively limited to begin with. Theoretically, increases in drug-enforcement efforts should result in reduced availability, higher prices, and lower purity of illegal drugs. That is, in fact, what has happened to the domestic marijuana market (in at least the first two respects). But in general the illegal drug market has not responded as intended to the substantial increases in federal, state, and local drug-enforcement efforts.

Cocaine has sold for about a hundred dollars a gram at the retail level since the beginning of the 1980s. The average purity of that gram, however, has increased from 12 to 60 percent. Moreover, a growing number of users are turning to "crack," a potent derivative of cocaine that can be smoked; it is widely sold in ghetto neighborhoods now for five to ten dollars per vial. Needless to say, both crack and the 60 percent pure cocaine pose much greater threats to users than did the relatively benign powder available eight years ago. Similarly, the retail price of heroin has remained relatively constant even as the average purity has risen from 3.9 percent in 1983 to 6.1 percent in 1986. Throughout the southwestern part of the United States, a particularly potent form of heroin known as "black tar" has become increasingly prevalent. And in many cities, a powerful synthetic opiate, Dilaudid, is beginning to compete with heroin as the preferred opiate. The growing number of heroin-related hospital emergencies and deaths is directly related to these developments.

All of these trends suggest that drug-enforcement efforts are not succeeding and may even be backfiring. There are numerous indications, for instance, that a growing number of marijuana dealers in both the producer countries and the United States are switching to cocaine dealing, motivated both by the promise of greater profits and by government drug-enforcement efforts that place a premium on minimizing the bulk of the illicit product (in order to avoid detection). It is possible, of course, that some of these trends would be even more severe in the absence of drug laws and enforcement. At the same time, it is worth observing that the increases in the potency of illegal drugs have coincided with decreases in the potency of legal substances. Motivated in good part by health concerns, cigarette smokers are turning increasingly to lower-tar and lower-nicotine tobacco products, alcohol drinkers from hard liquor to wine and beer, and even coffee drinkers from regular to decaffeinated coffee. This trend may well have less to do with the nature of the substances than with their legal status. It is quite possible, for instance, that the subculture of illicit-drug use creates a bias or incentive in favor of riskier behavior and more powerful psychoactive effects. If this is the case, legalization might well succeed in reversing today's trend toward more potent drugs and more dangerous methods of consumption.

The most "successful" drug-enforcement operations are those that succeed in identifying and destroying an entire drug-trafficking organization. Such operations can send dozens of people to jail and earn the government millions of dollars in asset forfeitures. Yet these operations have virtually no effect on the availability or price of illegal drugs throughout much of the United States. During the past few years, some urban police departments have devoted

18

significant manpower and financial resources to intensive crack-downs on street-level drug dealing in particular neighborhoods. Code-named Operation Pressure Point, Operation Clean Sweep, and so on, these massive police efforts have led to hundreds, even thousands, of arrests of low-level dealers and drug users and have helped improve the quality of life in the targeted neighborhoods. In most cases, however, drug dealers have adapted relatively easily by moving their operations to nearby neighborhoods. In the final analysis, the principal accomplishment of most domestic drug-enforcement efforts is not to reduce the supply or availability of illegal drugs, or even to raise their price; it is to punish the drug dealers who are apprehended, and cause minor disruptions in established drug markets.

The Failure of International Drug Control

Many drug-enforcement officials and urban leaders recognize the futility of domestic drug-enforcement efforts and place their hopes in international control efforts. Yet these too are doomed to fail—for numerous reasons. First, marijuana and opium can be grown almost anywhere, and the coca plant, from which cocaine is derived, is increasingly being cultivated successfully in areas that were once considered inhospitable environments. Wherever drug-eradication efforts succeed, other regions and countries are quick to fill the void; for example, Colombian marijuana growers rapidly expanded production following successful eradication efforts in Mexico during the mid-1970s. Today, Mexican growers are rapidly taking advantage of recent Colombian government successes in eradicating marijuana in the Guajira peninsula. Meanwhile, Jamaicans and Central Americans from Panama to Belize, as well as a growing assortment of Asians and Africans, do what they can to sell their own marijuana in American markets. And within the United States, domestic marijuana production is believed to be a multi-billion-dollar industry, supplying between 15 and 50 percent of the American market.

This push-down/pop-up factor also characterizes the international heroin market. At various points during the past two decades, Turkey, Mexico, Southeast Asia (Burma, Thailand, and Laos), and Southwest Asia (Pakistan, Afghanistan, and Iran) have each served as the principal source of heroin imported into the

United States. During the early 1970s, Mexican producers rapidly filled the void created by the Turkish government's successful opium-control measures. Although a successful eradication program during the latter part of the 1970s reduced Mexico's share of the U.S. market from a peak of 87 percent in 1975, it has since retained at least a one-third share in each year. Southwest Asian producers, who had played no role in supplying the American market as late as 1976, were able to supply over half the American market four years later. Today, increasing evidence indicates that drug traffickers are bringing unprecedented quantities of Southeast Asian heroin into the United States.

So far, the push-down/pop-up factor has played little role in the international cocaine market, for the simple reason that no government has yet pushed down in a significant way. Unlike marijuana- and opium-eradication efforts, in which aerial spraying of herbicides plays a prominent role, coca-eradication efforts are still conducted manually. The long-anticipated development and approval of an environmentally safe herbicide to destroy coca plants may introduce an unprecedented push-down factor into the market. But even in the absence of such government pressures, coca growing has expanded rapidly during the past decade within Bolivia and Peru, and has expanded outward into Colombia, Brazil, Ecuador, Venezuela, and elsewhere. Moreover, once eradication efforts do begin, coca growers can be expected to adopt many of the same "guerrilla farming" methods adopted by marijuana and opium growers to camouflage and protect their crops from eradication efforts.

Beyond the push-down/pop-up factor, international source-control efforts face a variety of other obstacles. In many countries, governments with limited resources lack the ability to crack down on drug production in the hinterlands and other poorly policed regions. In some countries, ranging from Colombia and Peru to Burma and Thailand, leftist insurgencies are involved in drug production for either financial or political profit and may play an important role in hampering government drug-control efforts. With respect to all three of the illicit crops, poor peasants with no comparable opportunites to earn as much money growing legitimate produce are prominently involved in the illicit business. In some cases, the illicit crop is part of a traditional, indigenous culture. Even where it is not, peasants typically perceive little or nothing immoral about taking advantage of the opportunity to grow the illicit crops. Indeed, from their perspective their moral obligation is not to protect the foolish American consumer of their produce but to provide for their families' welfare. And even among those who do perceive participation in the illicit drug market as somewhat unethical, the temptations held out by the drug traffickers often prove overwhelming.

No illicit drug is as difficult to keep out of the United States as heroin. The absence of geographical limitations on where it can be cultivated is just one minor obstacle. American heroin users consume an estimated 6 tons of heroin each year. The 60 tons of opium required to produce that heroin represent just 2 or 3 percent of the estimated 2,000 to 3,000 tons of illicit opium produced during each of the past few years. Even if eradication efforts combined with what often proves to be the opium growers' principal nemesis—bad weather—were to eliminate three-fourths of that production in one year, the U.S. market would still require just 10 percent of the remaining crop. Since U.S. consumers are able and willing to pay more than any others, the chances are good that they would still obtain their heroin. In any event, the prospects for such a radical reduction in illicit opium production are scanty indeed.

As Peter Reuter argues,[1] interdiction, like source control, is largely unable to keep illicit drugs out of the United States. Moreover, the past twenty years' experience has demonstrated that even dramatic increases in interdiction and source-control efforts have little or no effect on the price and purity of drugs. The few small successes, such as the destruction of the Turkish-opium "French Connection" in the early 1970s and the crackdown on Mexican marijuana and heroin in the late 1970s, were exceptions to the rule. The elusive goal of international drug control since then has been to replicate those unusual successes. It is a strategy that is destined to fail, however, as long as millions of Americans continue to demand the illicit substances that foreigners are willing and able to supply.

[1] Peter Reuter, "Can the Borders Be Sealed?" *Public Interest* 92 (Summer 1988): 51–65.

The Costs of Prohibition

The fact that drug-prohibition laws and policies cannot eradicate or even significantly reduce drug abuse is not necessarily a reason to repeal them. They do, after all, succeed in deterring many people from trying drugs, and they clearly reduce the availability and significantly increase the price of illegal drugs. These accomplishments alone might warrant retaining the drug laws, were it not for the fact that these same laws are also responsible for much of what Americans identify as the "drug problem." Here the analogies to alcohol and tobacco are worth noting. There is little question that we could reduce the health costs associated with use and abuse of alcohol and tobacco if we were to criminalize their production, sale, and possession. But no one believes that we could eliminate their use and abuse, that we could create an "alcohol-free" or "tobacco-free" country. Nor do most Americans believe that criminalizing the alcohol and tobacco markets would be a good idea. Their opposition stems largely from two beliefs: that adult Americans have the right to choose what substances they will consume and what risks they will take and that the costs of trying to coerce so many Americans to abstain from those substances would be enormous. It was the strength of these two beliefs that ultimately led to the repeal of Prohibition, and it is partly due to memories of that experience that criminalizing either alcohol or tobacco has little support today.

Consider the potential consequences of criminalizing the production, sale, and possession of all tobacco products. On the positive side, the number of people smoking tobacco would almost certainly decline, as would the health costs associated with tobacco consumption. Although the "forbidden fruit" syndrome would attract some people to cigarette smoking who would not otherwise have smoked, many more would likely be deterred by the criminal sanction, the moral standing of the law, the higher cost and unreliable quality of the illicit tobacco, and the difficulties involved in acquiring it. Non-smokers would rarely if ever be bothered by the irritating habits of their fellow citizens. The anti-tobacco laws would discourage some people from ever starting to smoke and would induce others to quit.

On the negative side, however, millions of Americans, including both tobacco addicts and recreational users, would no doubt defy the law, generating a massive underground market and billions in profits for organized criminals. Although some tobacco farmers would find other work, thousands more would become outlaws and continue to produce their crops covertly. Throughout Latin America, farmers and gangsters would rejoice at the opportunity to earn untold sums of gringo greenbacks, even as U.S. diplomats pressured foreign governments to cooperate with U.S. laws. Within the United States, government helicopters would spray herbicides on illicit tobacco fields; people would be rewarded by the government for informing on their neighbors who grow, sell, and smoke tobacco; urine tests would be employed to identify violators of the anti-tobacco laws; and a Tobacco Enforcement Administration (the T.E.A.) would employ undercover agents, informants, and wiretaps to uncover tobacco-law violators. Municipal, state, and federal judicial systems would be clogged with tobacco traffickers and "abusers." "Tobacco-related murders" would increase dramatically as criminal organizations competed with one another for turf and markets. Smoking would become an act of youthful rebellion, and no doubt some users would begin to experiment with more concentrated, potent, and dangerous forms of tobacco. Tobacco-related corruption would infect all levels of government, and respect for the law would decline noticeably. Government expenditures on tobacco-law enforcement would climb rapidly into the billions of dollars, even as budget balancers longingly recalled the almost ten billion dollars per year in tobacco taxes earned by the federal and state governments prior to prohibition. Finally, the state of North Carolina might even secede again from the Union.

This seemingly far-fetched tobacco-prohibition scenario is little more than an extrapolation based on the current situation with respect to marijuana, cocaine, and heroin. In many ways, our predicament resembles what actually happened during Prohibition. Prior to Prohibition, most Americans hoped that alcohol could be effectively banned by passing laws against its production and supply. During the early years of Prohibition, when drinking declined but millions of Americans nonetheless continued to drink, Prohibition's supporters placed their faith in tougher laws and more police and jails. After a few more years, however, increasing numbers of Americans began to realize that laws and policemen were unable to eliminate the smugglers, bootleggers, and illicit producers, as long as tens of millions of Americans continued to want to buy alcohol. At the same time, they saw that more laws and police-men seemed to generate more violence and corruption, more crowded courts and jails, wider disrespect for government and the law, and more power and profits for the gangsters. Repeal of Prohibition came to be seen not as a capitulation to Al Capone and his ilk but as a means of both putting the bootleggers out of business and eliminating most of the costs associated with the prohibition laws.

Today, Americans are faced with a dilemma similar to that con-fronted by our forebears sixty years ago. Demand for illicit drugs shows some signs of abating but no signs of declining significantly. Moreover, there are substantial reasons to doubt that tougher laws and policing have played an important role in reducing consump-tion. Supply, meanwhile, has not abated at all. Availability of illicit drugs, except for marijuana in some locales, remains high. Prices are dropping, even as potency increases. And the number of drug producers, smugglers, and dealers remains sizable, even as jails and prisons fill to overflowing. As was the case during Prohibition, the principal beneficiaries of current drug policies are the new and old organized-crime gangs. The principal victims, on the other hand, are not the drug dealers but the tens of millions of Americans who are worse off in one way or another as a consequence of the existence and failure of the drug-prohibition laws.

All public policies create beneficiaries and victims, both intended and unintended. When a public policy results in a disproportionate magnitude of unintended victims, there is good reason to reevalu-ate the assumptions and design of the policy. In the case of drug-prohibition policies, the intended beneficiaries are those individuals who would become drug abusers but for the existence and enforce-ment of the drug laws. The intended victims are those who traffic in illicit drugs and suffer the legal consequences. The unintended beneficiaries, conversely, are the drug producers and traffickers who profit handsomely from the illegality of the market, while avoiding arrest by the authorities and the violence perpetrated by other criminals. The unintended victims of drug-prohibition policies are rarely recognized as such, however. Viewed narrowly, they are the thirty million Americans who use illegal drugs, thereby risking loss of their jobs, imprisonment, and the damage done to health by ingesting illegally produced drugs; viewed broadly, they

24

are all Americans, who pay the substantial costs of our present ill-considered policies, both as taxpayers and as the potential victims of crime. These unintended victims are generally thought to be victimized by the unintended beneficiaries (i.e., the drug dealers), when in fact it is the drug-prohibition policies themselves that are primarily responsible for their plight.

If law-enforcement efforts could succeed in significantly reducing either the supply of illicit drugs or the demand for them, we would probably have little need to seek alternative drug-control policies. But since those efforts have repeatedly failed to make much of a difference and show little indication of working better in the future, at this point we must focus greater attention on their costs. Unlike the demand and supply of illicit drugs, which have remained relatively indifferent to legislative initiatives, the costs of drug-enforcement measures can be affected—quite dramatically—by legislative measures. What tougher criminal sanctions and more police have failed to accomplish, in terms of reducing drug-related violence, corruption, death, and social decay, may well be better accomplished by legislative repeal of the drug laws and adoption of less punitive but more effective measures to prevent and treat substance abuse.

Costs to the Taxpayer

Since 1981, federal expenditures on drug enforcement have more than tripled—from less than one billion dollars a year to about three billion. According to the National Drug Enforcement Policy Board, the annual budgets of the Drug Enforcement Administration (DEA) and the Coast Guard have each risen during the past seven years from about $220 million to roughly $500 million. During the same period, FBI resources devoted to drug enforcement have increased from $8 million a year to over $100 million, U.S. Marshals resources from $26 million to about $80 million, U.S. Attorney resources from $20 million to about $100 million, State Department resources from $35 million to $100 million, U.S. Customs resources from $180 million to over $400 million, and Bureau of Prison resources from $77 million to about $300 million. Expenditures on drug control by the military and the intelligence agencies are more difficult to calculate, although by all accounts they have increased by at least the same magnitude and now total hundreds of millions of dollars per year. Even greater are the expenditures at lower levels of government. In a 1987 study for the U.S. Customs Service by Wharton Econometrics, state and local police were estimated to have devoted 18 percent of their total investigative resources, or close to five billion dollars, to drug-enforcement activities in 1986. This represented a 19 percent increase over the previous year's expenditures. All told, 1987 expenditures on all aspects of drug enforcement, from drug eradication in foreign countries to imprisonment of drug users and dealers in the United States, totaled at least ten billion dollars.

Of course, even ten billion dollars a year pales in comparison with expenditures on military defense. Of greater concern than the actual expenditures, however, has been the diversion of limited resources—including the time and energy of judges, prosecutors, and law-enforcement agents, as well as scarce prison space—from the prosecution and punishment of criminal activities that harm far more innocent victims than do violations of the drug laws. Drug-law violators account for approximately 10 percent of the roughly 800,000 inmates in state prisons and local jails and more than one-third of the 44,000 federal prison inmates. These proportions are expected to increase in coming years, even as total prison populations continue to rise dramatically.[2] Among the 40,000 inmates in New York State prisons, drug-law violations surpassed first-degree robbery in 1987 as the number one cause of incarceration, accounting for 20 percent of the total prison population. The U.S. Sentencing Commission has estimated that, largely as a consequence of the Anti-Drug Act passed by Congress in 1986, the proportion of federal inmates incarcerated for drug violations will rise from one-third of the 44,000 prisoners sentenced to federal-prison terms today to one-half of the 100,000 to 150,000 federal prisoners anticipated in fifteen years. The direct costs of building and maintaining enough prisons to house this growing population are rising at an astronomical rate. The opportunity costs, in terms of alternative social expenditures

[2]The total number of state and federal prison inmates in 1975 was under 250,000; in 1980 it was 350,000; and in 1987 it was 575,000. The projected total for 2000 is one million. See John J. DiIulio, Jr., "What's Wrong with Private Prisons," *Public Interest* 92 (Summer 1988): 66–83.

forgone and other types of criminals not imprisoned, are perhaps even greater.[3]

During each of the last few years, police made about 750,000 arrests for violations of the drug laws. Slightly more than three-quarters of these have not been for manufacturing or dealing drugs but solely for possession of an illicit drug, typically marijuana. (Those arrested, it is worth noting, represent little more than 2 percent of the thirty million Americans estimated to have used an illegal drug during the past year.) On the one hand, this has clogged many urban criminal-justice systems: in New York City, drug-law violations last year accounted for more than 40 percent of all felony indictments—up from 25 percent in 1985; in Washington, D.C., the figure was more than 50 percent. On the other hand, it has distracted criminal-justice officials from concentrating greater resources on violent offenses and property crimes. In many cities, law enforcement has become virtually synonymous with drug enforcement.

Drug laws typically have two effects on the market in illicit drugs. The first is to restrict the general availability and accessibility of illicit drugs, especially in locales where underground drug markets are small and isolated from the community. The second is to increase, often significantly, the price of illicit drugs to consumers. Since the costs of producing most illicit drugs are not much different from the costs of alcohol, tobacco, and coffee, most of the price paid for illicit substances is in effect a value-added tax created by their criminalization, which is enforced and supplemented by the law-enforcement establishment but collected by the drug traffickers. A report by Wharton Econometrics for the President's Commission on Organized Crime identified the sale of illicit drugs as the source of more than half of all organized-crime revenues in 1986, with the marijuana and heroin business each providing over seven billion dollars and the cocaine business over thirteen billion. By contrast, revenues from cigarette bootlegging, which persists principally because of differences among the states in their cigarette-tax rates, were estimated at 290 million dollars. If the marijuana, cocaine, and

[3]It should be emphasized that the numbers cited do not include the many inmates sentenced for "drug-related" crimes such as acts of violence committed by drug dealers, typically against one another, and robberies committed to earn the money needed to pay for illegal drugs.

heroin markets were legal, state and federal governments would collect billions of dollars annually in tax revenues. Instead, they expend billions on what amounts to a subsidy of organized crime and unorganized criminals.

Drugs and Crime

The drug/crime connection is one that continues to resist coherent analysis, both because cause and effect are so difficult to distinguish and because the role of the drug-prohibition laws in causing and labeling "drug-related crime" is so often ignored. There are four possible connections between drugs and crime, at least three of which would be much diminished if the drug-prohibition laws were repealed. First, producing, selling, buying, and consuming strictly controlled and banned substances are crimes that occur billions of times each year in the United States alone. In the absence of drug-prohibition laws, these activities would obviously cease to be crimes. Selling drugs to children would, of course, continue to be criminal, and other evasions of government regulation of a legal market would continue to be prosecuted; but by and large the drug/crime connection that now accounts for all of the criminal-justice costs noted above would be severed.

Second, many illicit-drug users commit crimes such as robbery and burglary, as well as drug dealing, prostitution, and numbers running, to earn enough money to purchase the relatively high-priced illicit drugs. Unlike the millions of alcoholics who can support their habits for relatively modest amounts, many cocaine and heroin addicts spend hundreds and even thousands of dollars a week. If the drugs to which they are addicted were significantly cheaper—which would be the case if they were legalized—the number of crimes committed by drug addicts to pay for their habits would, in all likelihood, decline dramatically. Even if a legal-drug policy included the imposition of relatively high consumption taxes in order to discourage consumption, drug prices would probably still be lower than they are today.

The third drug/crime connection is the commission of crimes—violent crimes in particular—by people under the influence of illicit drugs. This connection seems to have the greatest impact upon the popular imagination. Clearly, some drugs do "cause" some people to commit crimes by reducing normal inhibitions, unleashing

28

aggressive and other anti-social tendencies, and lessening the sense of responsibility. Cocaine, particularly in the form of crack, has gained such a reputation in recent years, just as heroin did in the 1960s and 1970s and marijuana did in the years before that. Crack's reputation for inspiring violent behavior may or may not be more deserved than those of marijuana and heroin; reliable evidence is not yet available. No illicit drug, however, is as widely associated with violent behavior as alcohol. According to Justice Department statistics, 54 percent of all jail inmates convicted of violent crimes in 1983 reported having used alcohol just prior to committing their offense. The impact of drug legalization on this drug/crime connection is the most difficult to predict. Much would depend on overall rates of drug abuse and changes in the nature of consumption, both of which are impossible to predict. It is worth noting, however, that a shift in consumption from alcohol to marijuana would almost certainly contribute to a decline in violent behavior.

The fourth drug/crime link is the violent, intimidating, and corrupting behavior of the drug traffickers. Illegal markets tend to breed violence—not only because they attract criminally minded individuals but also because participants in the market have no resort to legal institutions to resolve their disputes. During Prohibition, violent struggles between bootlegging gangs and hijackings of booze-laden trucks and sea vessels were frequent and notorious occurrences. Today's equivalents are the booby traps that surround some marijuana fields, the pirates of the Caribbean looking to rip off drug-laden vessels en route to the shores of the United States, and the machine-gun battles and executions carried out by drug lords—all of which occasionally kill innocent people. Most law-enforcement officials agree that the dramatic increases in urban murder rates during the past few years can be explained almost entirely by the rise in drug-dealer killings.

Perhaps the most unfortunate victims of the drug-prohibition policies have been the law-abiding residents of America's ghettos. These policies have largely proven futile in deterring large numbers of ghetto dwellers from becoming drug abusers, but they do account for much of what ghetto residents identify as the drug problem. In many neighborhoods, it often seems to be the aggressive gun-toting drug dealers who upset law-abiding residents far more than the addicts nodding out in doorways. Other residents, however, perceive the drug dealers as heroes and successful role models. In

29

impoverished neighborhoods, they often stand out as symbols of success to children who see no other options. At the same time, the increasingly harsh criminal penalties imposed on adult drug dealers have led to the widespread recruitment of juveniles by drug traffickers. Formerly, children started dealing drugs only after they had been using them for a while; today the sequence is often reversed: many children start using illegal drugs now only after working for older drug dealers. And the juvenile-justice system offers no realistic options for dealing with this growing problem.

The conspicuous failure of law-enforcement agencies to deal with this drug/crime connection is probably most responsible for the demoralization of neighborhoods and police departments alike. Intensive police crackdowns in urban neighborhoods do little more than chase the menace a short distance away to infect new areas. By contrast, legalization of the drug market would drive the drug-dealing business off the streets and out of apartment buildings and into legal, government-regulated, tax-paying stores. It would also force many of the gun-toting dealers out of business and would convert others into legitimate businessmen. Some, of course, would turn to other types of criminal activities, just as some of the bootleggers did following Prohibition's repeal. Gone, however, would be the unparalleled financial temptations that lure so many people from all sectors of society into the drug-dealing business.

The Costs of Corruption

All vice-control efforts are particularly susceptible to corruption, but none so much as drug enforcement. When police accept bribes from drug dealers, no victim exists to complain to the authorities. Even when police extort money and drugs from traffickers and dealers, the latter are in no position to report the corrupt officers. What makes drug enforcement especially vulnerable to corruption are the tremendous amounts of money involved in the business. Today, many law-enforcement officials believe that police corruption is more pervasive than at any time since Prohibition. In Miami, dozens of law-enforcement officials have been charged with accepting bribes, stealing from drug dealers, and even dealing drugs themselves. Throughout many small towns and rural communities in Georgia, where drug smugglers en route from Mexico, the Caribbean, and Latin America drop their loads of cocaine and marijuana, dozens of sheriffs have been implicated in drug-related corruption. In New York, drug-related corruption in one Brooklyn police precinct has generated the city's most far-reaching police-corruption scandal since the 1960s. More than a hundred cases of drug-related corruption are now prosecuted each year in state and federal courts. Every one of the federal law-enforcement agencies charged with drug-enforcement responsibilities has seen an agent implicated in drug-related corruption.

It is not difficult to explain the growing pervasiveness of drug-related corruption. The financial temptations are enormous relative to other opportunities, legitimate or illegitimate. Little effort is required. Many police officers are demoralized by the scope of the drug traffic, their sense that many citizens are indifferent, and the fact that many sectors of society do not even appreciate their efforts—as well as the fact that many of the drug dealers who are arrested do not remain in prison. Some police also recognize that enforcing the drug laws does not protect victims from predators so much as it regulates an illicit market that cannot be suppressed but can be kept underground. In every respect, the analogy to Prohibition is apt. Repealing the drug-prohibition laws would dramatically reduce police corruption. By contrast, the measures currently being proposed to deal with the growing problem, including better funded and more aggressive internal investigations, offer relatively little promise.

Among the most difficult costs to evaluate are those that relate to the widespread defiance of the drug-prohibition laws: the effects of labeling as criminals the tens of millions of people who use drugs illicitly, subjecting them to the risks of criminal sanction, and obligating many of these same people to enter into relationships with drug dealers (who may be criminals in many more senses of the word) in order to purchase their drugs; the cynicism that such laws generate toward other laws and the law in general; and the sense of hostility and suspicion that many otherwise law-abiding individuals feel toward law-enforcement officials. It was costs such as these that strongly influenced many of Prohibition's more conservative opponents.

Physical and Moral Costs

Perhaps the most paradoxical consequence of the drug laws is the tremendous harm they cause to the millions of drug users who

31

have not been deterred from using illicit drugs in the first place. Nothing resembling an underground Food and Drug Administration has arisen to impose quality control on the illegal drug market and provide users with accurate information on the drugs they consume. Imagine that Americans could not tell whether a bottle of wine contained 6 percent, 30 percent, or 90 percent alcohol, or whether an aspirin tablet contained 5 or 500 grams of aspirin. Imagine, too, that no controls existed to prevent winemakers from diluting their product with methanol and other dangerous impurities and that vineyards and tobacco fields were fertilized with harmful substances by ignorant growers and sprayed with poisonous herbicides by government agents. Fewer people would use such substances, but more of those who did would get sick. Some would die.

The above scenario describes, of course, the current state of the illicit drug market. Many marijuana smokers are worse off for having smoked cannabis that was grown with dangerous fertilizers, sprayed with the herbicide paraquat, or mixed with more dangerous substances. Consumers of heroin and the various synthetic substances sold on the street face even severer consequences, including fatal overdoses and poisonings from unexpectedly potent or impure drug supplies. More often than not, the quality of a drug addict's life depends greatly upon his or her access to reliable supplies. Drug-enforcement operations that succeed in temporarily disrupting supply networks are thus a double-edged sword: they encourage some addicts to seek admission into drug-treatment programs, but they oblige others to seek out new and hence less reliable suppliers; the result is that more, not fewer, drug-related emergencies and deaths occur.

Today, over 50 percent of all people with AIDS in New York City, New Jersey, and many other parts of the country, as well as the vast majority of AIDS-infected heterosexuals throughout the country, have contracted the disease directly or indirectly through illegal intravenous drug use. Reports have emerged of drug dealers' beginning to provide clean syringes together with their illegal drugs. But even as other governments around the world actively attempt to limit the spread of AIDS by and among drug users by instituting free syringe-exchange programs, state and municipal governments in the United States resist following suit, arguing that to do so would "encourage" or "condone" the use of illegal drugs. Only in January 1988 did New York City approve such a program on a very limited and experimental basis. At the same time, drug-treatment programs remain notoriously underfunded, turning away tens of thousands of addicts seeking help, even as billions of dollars more are spent to arrest, prosecute, and imprison illegal drug sellers and users. In what may represent a sign of shifting priorities, the President's Commission on AIDS, in its March 1988 report, emphasized the importance of making drug-treatment programs available to all in need of them. In all likelihood, however, the criminal-justice agencies will continue to receive the greatest share of drug-control funds.

Most Americans perceive the drug problem as a moral issue and draw a moral distinction between use of the illicit drugs and use of alcohol and tobacco. Yet when one subjects this distinction to reasoned analysis, it quickly disintegrates. The most consistent moral perspective of those who favor drug laws is that of the Mormons and the Puritans, who regard as immoral any intake of substances to alter one's state of consciousness or otherwise cause pleasure: they forbid not only the illicit drugs and alcohol but also tobacco, caffeine, and even chocolate. The vast majority of Americans are hardly so consistent with respect to the propriety of their pleasures. Yet once one acknowledges that there is nothing immoral about drinking alcohol or smoking tobacco for non-medicinal purposes, it becomes difficult to condemn the consumption of marijuana, cocaine, and other substances on moral grounds. The "moral" condemnation of some substances and not others proves to be little more than a prejudice in favor of some drugs and against others.

The same false distinction is drawn with respect to those who provide the psychoactive substances to users and abusers alike. If degrees of immorality were measured by the levels of harm caused by one's products, the "traffickers" in tobacco and alcohol would be vilified as the most evil of all substance purveyors. That they are perceived instead as respected members of our community, while providers of the no more dangerous illicit substances are punished with long prison sentences, says much about the prejudices of most Americans with respect to psychoactive substances but little about the morality or immorality of purveyors' activities.

Much the same is true of gun salesmen. Most of the consumers of their products use them safely; a minority, however, end up shooting either themselves or someone else. Can we hold the gun salesman morally culpable for the harm that probably would not have occurred but for his existence? Most people say no, except perhaps where the salesman clearly knew that his product would be used to commit a crime. Yet in the case of those who sell illicit substances to willing customers, the providers are deemed not only legally guilty but also morally reprehensible. The law does not require any demonstration that the dealer knew of a specific harm to follow; indeed, it does not require any evidence at all of harm having resulted from the sale. Rather, the law is predicated on the assumption that harm will inevitably follow. Despite the patent falsity of that assumption, it persists as the underlying justification for the drug laws.

Although a valid moral distinction cannot be drawn between the licit and the illicit psychoactive substances, one can point to a different kind of moral justification for the drug laws: they arguably reflect a paternalistic obligation to protect those in danger of succumbing to their own weaknesses. If drugs were legally available, most people would either abstain from using them or would use them responsibly and in moderation. A minority without self-restraint, however, would end up harming themselves if the substances were more readily available. Therefore, the majority has a moral obligation to deny itself legal access to certain substances because of the plight of the minority. This obligation is presumably greatest when children are included among the minority.

At least in principle, this argument seems to provide the strongest moral justification for the drug laws. But ultimately the moral quality of laws must be judged not by how those laws are intended to work in principle but by how they function in practice. When laws intended to serve a moral end inflict great damage on innocent parties, we must rethink our moral position.

Because drug-law violations do not create victims with an interest in notifying the police, drug-enforcement agents rely heavily on undercover operations, electronic surveillance, and information provided by informants. These techniques are indispensable to effective law enforcement, but they are also among the least palatable investigative methods employed by the police. The same is true of drug testing: it may be useful and even necessary for determining liability in accidents, but it also threatens and undermines the right of privacy to which many Americans believe they are entitled. There are good reasons for requiring that such measures be used sparingly.

Equally disturbing are the increasingly vocal calls for people to inform not only on drug dealers but also on neighbors, friends, and even family members who use illicit drugs. Government calls on people not only to "just say no" but also to report those who have not heeded the message. Intolerance of illicit-drug use and users is heralded not only as an indispensable ingredient in the war against drugs but also as a mark of good citizenship. Certainly every society requires citizens to assist in the enforcement of criminal laws. But societies—particularly democratic and pluralistic ones—also rely strongly on an ethic of tolerance toward those who are different but do no harm to others. Overzealous enforcement of the drug laws risks undermining that ethic and encouraging the creation of a society of informants. This results in an immorality that is far more dangerous in its own way than that associated with the use of illicit drugs.

The Benefits of Legalization

Repealing the drug-prohibition laws promises tremendous advantages. Between reduced government expenditures on enforcing drug laws and new tax revenue from legal drug production and sales, public treasuries would enjoy a net benefit of at least ten billion dollars a year, and possibly much more. The quality of urban life would rise significantly. Homicide rates would decline. So would robbery and burglary rates. Organized criminal groups, particularly the newer ones that have yet to diversify out of drugs, would be dealt a devastating setback. The police, prosecutors, and courts would focus their resources on combatting the types of crimes that people cannot walk away from. More ghetto residents would turn their backs on criminal careers and seek out legitimate opportunities instead. And the health and quality of life of many drug users—and even drug abusers—would improve significantly.

All the benefits of legalization would be for naught, however, if millions more Americans were to become drug abusers. Our experience with alcohol and tobacco provides ample warnings.

35

Today, alcohol is consumed by 140 million Americans and tobacco by 50 million. All of the health costs associated with abuse of the illicit drugs pale in comparison with those resulting from tobacco and alcohol abuse. In 1986, for example, alcohol was identified as a contributing factor in 10 percent of work-related injuries, 40 percent of suicide attempts, and about 40 percent of the approximately 46,000 annual traffic deaths in 1983. An estimated eighteen million Americans are reported to be either alcoholics or alcohol abusers. The total cost of alcohol abuse to American society is estimated at over 100 billion dollars annually. Alcohol has been identified as the direct cause of 80,000 to 100,000 deaths annually and as a contributing factor in an additional 100,000 deaths. The health costs of tobacco use are of similar magnitude. In the United States alone, an estimated 320,000 people die prematurely each year as a consequence of their consumption of tobacco. By comparison, the National Council on Alcoholism reported that only 3,562 people were known to have died in 1985 from use of all illegal drugs combined. Even if we assume that thousands more deaths were related in one way or another to illicit drug abuse but not reported as such, we are still left with the conclusion that all of the health costs of marijuana, cocaine, and heroin combined amount to only a small fraction of those caused by tobacco and alcohol.

Most Americans are just beginning to recognize the extensive costs of alcohol and tobacco abuse. At the same time, they seem to believe that there is something fundamentally different about alcohol and tobacco that supports the legal distinction between those two substances, on the one hand, and the illicit ones, on the other. The most common distinction is based on the assumption that the illicit drugs are more dangerous than the licit ones. Cocaine, heroin, the various hallucinogens, and (to a lesser extent) marijuana are widely perceived as, in the words of the President's Commission on Organized Crime, "inherently destructive to mind and body." They are also believed to be more addictive and more likely to cause dangerous and violent behavior than alcohol and tobacco. All use of illicit drugs is therefore thought to be abusive; in other words, the distinction between use and abuse of psychoactive substances that most people recognize with respect to alcohol is not acknowledged with respect to the illicit substances.

Most Americans make the fallacious assumption that the government would not criminalize certain psychoactive substances if they

36

were not in fact dangerous. Then they jump to the conclusion that any use of those substances is a form of abuse. The government, in its effort to discourage people from using illicit drugs, has encouraged and perpetuated these misconceptions—not only in its rhetoric but also in its purportedly educational materials. Only by reading between the lines can one discern the fact that the vast majority of Americans who have used illicit drugs have done so in moderation, that relatively few have suffered negative short-term consequences, and that few are likely to suffer long-term harm.

The evidence is most persuasive with respect to marijuana. U.S. drug-enforcement and health agencies do not even report figures on marijuana-related deaths, apparently because so few occur. Although there are good health reasons for children, pregnant women, and some others not to smoke marijuana, there still appears to be little evidence that occasional marijuana consumption does much harm. Certainly, it is not healthy to inhale marijuana smoke into one's lungs; indeed, the National Institute on Drug Abuse (NIDA) has declared that "marijuana smoke contains more cancer-causing agents than are found in tobacco smoke." On the other hand, the number of joints smoked by all but a very small percentage of marijuana smokers is a tiny fraction of the twenty cigarettes a day smoked by the average cigarette smoker; indeed, the average may be closer to one or two joints a week than one or two a day. Note that NIDA defines a "heavy" marijuana smoker as one who consumes at least two joints "daily." A heavy tobacco smoker, by contrast, smokes about forty cigarettes a day.

Nor is marijuana strongly identified as a dependence-causing substance. A 1982 survey of marijuana use by young adults (eighteen to twenty-five years old) found that 64 percent had tried marijuana at least once, that 42 percent had used it at least ten times, and that 27 percent had smoked in the last month. It also found that 21 percent had passed through a period during which they smoked "daily" (defined as twenty or more days per month) but that only one-third of those currently smoked "daily" and only one-fifth (about 4 percent of all young adults) could be described as heavy daily users (averaging two or more joints per day). This suggests that daily marijuana use is typically a phase through which people pass, after which their use becomes more moderate.

Marijuana has also been attacked as the "gateway drug" that leads people to the use of even more dangerous illegal drugs. It is true that people who have smoked marijuana are more likely than people who have not to try, use, and abuse other illicit substances. It is also true that people who have smoked tobacco or drunk alcohol are more likely than those who have not to experiment with illicit drugs and to become substance abusers. The reasons are obvious enough. Familiarity with smoking cigarettes, for instance, removes one of the major barriers to smoking marijuana, which is the experience of inhaling smoke into one's lungs. Similarly, familiarity with altering one's state of consciousness by consuming psychoactive substances such as alcohol or marijuana decreases the fear and increases the curiosity regarding other substances and "highs." But the evidence also indicates that there is nothing inevitable about the process. The great majority of people who have smoked marijuana do not become substance abusers of either legal or illegal substances. At the same time, it is certainly true that many of those who do become substance abusers after using marijuana would have become abusers even if they had never smoked a joint in their lives.

Dealing with Drugs' Dangers

The dangers associated with cocaine, heroin, the hallucinogens, and other illicit substances are greater than those posed by marijuana, but not nearly so great as many people seem to think. Consider the case of cocaine. In 1986, NIDA reported that over 20 million Americans had tried cocaine, that 12.2 million had consumed it at least once during 1985, and that nearly 5.8 million had used it within the past month. Among those between the ages of eighteen and twenty-five, 8.2 million had tried cocaine, 5.3 million had used it within the past year, 2.5 million had used it within the past month, and 250,000 had used it weekly. Extrapolation might suggest that a quarter of a million young Americans are potential problem users. But one could also conclude that only 3 percent of those between the ages of eighteen and twenty-five who had ever tried the drug fell into that category and that only 10 percent of those who had used cocaine monthly were at risk. (The NIDA survey did not, it should be noted, include people residing in military or student dormitories, prison inmates, or the homeless.)

All of this is not to deny that cocaine is a potentially dangerous drug, especially when it is injected, smoked in the form of crack, or consumed in tandem with other powerful substances. Clearly, tens of thousands of Americans have suffered severely from their abuse of cocaine, and a tiny fraction have died. But there is also overwhelming evidence that most users of cocaine do not get into trouble with the drug. So much of the media attention has focused on the small percentage of cocaine users who become addicted that the popular perception of how most people use cocaine has become badly distorted. In one survey of high school seniors' drug use, the researchers questioned recent cocaine users, asking whether they had ever tried to stop using cocaine and found that they couldn't. Only 3.8 percent responded affirmatively, in contrast to the almost 7 percent of marijuana smokers who said they had tried to stop and found they couldn't and the 18 percent of cigarette smokers who answered similarly. Although a similar survey of adult users would probably reveal a higher proportion of cocaine addicts, evidence such as this suggests that only a small percentage of people who use cocaine end up having a problem with it. In this respect, most people differ from monkeys, who have demonstrated in experiments that they will starve themselves to death if provided with unlimited cocaine.

With respect to the hallucinogens such as LSD and psilocybic mushrooms, their potential for addiction is virtually nil. The dangers arise primarily from using them irresponsibly on individual occasions. Although many of those who have used one or another of the hallucinogens have experienced "bad trips," others have reported positive experiences, and very few have suffered any long-term harm.

Perhaps no drugs are regarded with as much horror as the opiates, and in particular heroin, which is a concentrated form of morphine. As with most drugs, heroin can be eaten, snorted, smoked, or injected. Most Americans, unfortunately, prefer injection. There is no question that heroin is potentially highly addictive, perhaps as addictive as nicotine. But despite the popular association of heroin use with the most down-and-out inhabitants of urban ghettos, heroin causes relatively little physical harm to the human body. Consumed on an occasional or regular basis under sanitary conditions, its worst side effect, apart from addiction itself, is constipation. That is one reason why many doctors in early twentieth-century America saw opiate addiction as preferable to alcoholism and prescribed the former as treatment for the latter when abstinence did not seem a realistic option.

It is important to think about the illicit drugs in the same way we think about alcohol and tobacco. Like tobacco, many of the illicit substances are highly addictive but can be consumed on a regular basis for decades without any demonstrable harm. Like alcohol, most of the substances can be, and are, used by most consumers in moderation, with little in the way of harmful effects; but like alcohol, they also lend themselves to abuse by a minority of users who become addicted or otherwise harm themselves or others as a consequence. And as is the case with both the legal substances, the psychoactive effects of the various illegal drugs vary greatly from one person to another. To be sure, the pharmacology of the substance is important, as are its purity and the manner in which it is consumed. But much also depends upon not only the physiology and psychology of the consumer but also his expectations regarding the drug, his social milieu, and the broader cultural environment—what Harvard University psychiatrist Norman Zinberg has called the "set and setting" of the drug. It is factors such as these that might change dramatically, albeit in indeterminate ways, were the illicit drugs made legally available.

Can Legalization Work?

It is thus impossible to predict whether legalization would lead to much greater levels of drug abuse and exact costs comparable to those of alcohol and tobacco abuse. The lessons that can be drawn from other societies are mixed. China's experience with the British opium pushers of the nineteenth century, when millions became addicted to the drug, offers one worst-case scenario. The devastation of many native American tribes by alcohol presents another. On the other hand, the legal availability of opium and cannabis in many Asian societies did not result in large addict populations until recently. Indeed, in many countries U.S.-inspired opium bans imposed during the past few decades have paradoxically contributed to dramatic increases in heroin consumption among Asian youth. Within the United States, the decriminalization of marijuana by about a dozen states during the 1970s did not lead to increases in marijuana consumption. In the Netherlands, which went even further in decriminalizing cannabis during the 1970s, consumption has actually declined significantly. The policy has succeeded, as the government intended, in making drug use boring. Finally, late nineteenth-century America was a society in which there were almost no drug laws or even drug regulations—but levels of drug use then were about what they are today. Drug abuse was considered a serious problem, but the criminal-justice system was not regarded as part of the solution.

There are, however, reasons to believe that none of the currently illicit substances would become as popular as alcohol or tobacco, even if they were legalized. Alcohol has long been the principal intoxicant in most societies, including many in which other substances have been legally available. Presumably, its diverse properties account for its popularity—it quenches thirst, goes well with food, and promotes appetite as well as sociability. The popularity of tobacco probably stems not just from its powerful addictive qualities but also from the fact that its psychoactive effects are sufficiently subtle that cigarettes can be integrated with most other human activities. The illicit substances do not share these qualities to the same extent, nor is it likely that they would acquire them if they were legalized. Moreover, none of the illicit substances can compete with alcohol's special place in American culture and history.

An additional advantage of the illicit drugs is that none of them appears to be as insidious as either alcohol or tobacco. Consumed in their more benign forms, few of the illicit substances are as damaging to the human body over the long term as alcohol and tobacco, and none is as strongly linked with violent behavior as alcohol. On the other hand, much of the damage caused today by illegal drugs stems from their consumption in particularly dangerous ways. There is good reason to doubt that many Americans would inject cocaine or heroin into their veins even if given the chance to do so legally. And just as the dramatic growth in the heroin-consuming population during the 1960s leveled off for reasons apparently having little to do with law enforcement, so we can expect a leveling off—which may already have begun—in the number of people smoking crack. The logic of legalization thus depends upon two assumptions: that most illegal drugs are not so dangerous as is commonly believed and that the drugs and methods of consumption that are most risky are unlikely to prove appealing to many people, precisely because they are so obviously dangerous.

Perhaps the most reassuring reason for believing that repeal of the drug-prohibition laws will not lead to tremendous increases in drug-abuse levels is the fact that we have learned something from our past experiences with alcohol and tobacco abuse. We now know, for instance, that consumption taxes are an effective method of limiting consumption rates. We also know that restrictions and bans on advertising, as well as a campaign of negative advertising, can make a difference. The same is true of other government measures, including restrictions on time and place of sale, prohibition of consumption in public places, packaging requirements, mandated adjustments in insurance policies, crackdowns on driving while under the influence, and laws holding bartenders and hosts responsible for the drinking of customers and guests. There is even some evidence that government-sponsored education programs about the dangers of cigarette smoking have deterred many children from beginning to smoke.

Clearly it is possible to avoid repeating the mistakes of the past in designing an effective plan for legalization. We know more about the illegal drugs now than we knew about alcohol when Prohibition was repealed or about tobacco when the anti-tobacco laws were repealed by many states in the early years of this century. Moreover, we can and must avoid having effective drug-control policies undermined by powerful lobbies like those that now protect the interests of alcohol and tobacco producers. We are also in a far better position than we were sixty years ago to prevent organized criminals from finding and creating new opportunities when their most lucrative source of income dries up.

It is important to stress what legalization is not. It is not a capitulation to the drug dealers—but rather a means to put them out of business. It is not an endorsement of drug use—but rather a recognition of the rights of adult Americans to make their own choices free of the fear of criminal sanctions. It is not a repudiation of the "just say no" approach—but rather an appeal to government to provide assistance and positive inducements, not criminal penalties and more repressive measures, in support of that approach. It is not even a call for the elimination of the criminal-justice system from drug regulation—but rather a proposal for the redirection of its efforts and attention.

There is no question that legalization is a risky policy, since it may lead to an increase in the number of people who abuse drugs.

But that is a risk—not a certainty. At the same time, current drug-control policies are failing, and new proposals promise only to be more costly and more repressive. We know that repealing the drug-prohibition laws would eliminate or greatly reduce many of the ills that people commonly identify as part and parcel of the "drug problem." Yet legalization is repeatedly and vociferously dismissed, without any attempt to evaluate it openly and objectively. The past twenty years have demonstrated that a drug policy shaped by exaggerated rhetoric designed to arouse fear has only led to our current disaster. Unless we are willing to honestly evaluate our options, including various legalization strategies, we will run a still greater risk: we may never find the best solution for our drug problems.

Thinking about Drug Legalization

James Ostrowski

> Prohibition is an awful flop.
> We like it.
> It can't stop what it's meant to stop.
> We like it.
> It's left a trail of graft and slime,
> It don't prohibit worth a dime,
> It's filled our land with vice and crime.
> Nevertheless, we're for it.
>
> Franklin P. Adams (1931)

On Thursday, March 17, 1988, at 10:45 p.m., in the Bronx, Vernia Brown was killed by stray bullets fired in a dispute over illegal drugs.[1] The 19-year-old mother of one was not involved in the dispute, yet her death was a direct consequence of the "war on drugs."

By now, there can be little doubt that most, if not all, "drug-related murders" are the result of drug prohibition. The same type of violence came with the Eighteenth Amendment's ban of alcohol in 1920. The murder rate rose with the start of Prohibition, remained high during Prohibition, and then declined for *11 consecutive years* when Prohibition ended.[2] The rate of assaults with a firearm rose

---

James Ostrowski is president of Citizens Against Prohibition.

This article is excerpted from "Thinking about Drug Legalization," Cato Institute Policy Analysis no. 121, May 25, 1989.

[1] *New York Times*, March 19, 1988, p. 29.

[2] The murder and assault rates had been rising even before Prohibition. Nevertheless, Prohibition's causal role in stimulating violence is indicated by the following facts: (1) the murder rate during Prohibition reached levels not surpassed until 1973, and (2) the rate declined sharply immediately after repeal. While there is apparently no comprehensive study of Prohibition-era violence, it is reported that there were more than 1,000 gangland murders in New York City alone during Prohibition. David E. Kyvig, *Repealing National Prohibition* (Chicago: University of Chicago Press, 1979), p. 27. Another writer estimates that 2,000 to 3,000 people died during law enforcement raids, auto chases, and arrests—casualties that by and large would not show up in murder statistics. Henry Lee, *How Dry We Were: Prohibition Revisited* (London: Prentice-Hall, 1963), p. 8.

with Prohibition and declined for *10 consecutive years* after Prohibition. In the last year of Prohibition—1933—there were 12,124 homicides and 7,863 assaults with firearms; by 1941 those figures had declined to 8,048 and 4,525, respectively.[3] (See Figure 1.)

Vernia Brown died because of the policy of drug prohibition. If her death was a "cost" of that policy, what did the "expenditure" of her life "buy"? What benefits has society derived from the policy of prohibition that led to her death? To find the answer, I turned to the experts and to the supporters of drug prohibition.

In 1988 I wrote to Vice President George Bush, then head of the South Florida Drug Task Force; to Education Secretary William Bennett; to Assistant Secretary of State for Drug Policy Ann Wrobleski; to White House drug policy adviser Dr. Donald I. McDonald; and to the public information directors of the Federal Bureau of Investigation, Drug Enforcement Administration, General Accounting Office, National Institute of Justice, and National Institute on Drug Abuse. None of those officials was able to cite any study that demonstrated the beneficial effects of drug prohibition weighed against its costs.

Some supporters of drug prohibition claim that its benefits are undeniable and self-evident. Their main assumption is that without prohibition drug use would skyrocket, with disastrous results. But there is little evidence for that commonly held belief. In fact, in the few cases where empirical evidence does exist it lends little support to the prediction of soaring drug use. For example, in two places in the Western world where use of small amounts of marijuana is legal—the Netherlands and Alaska—the rate of marijuana consumption is arguably *lower* than in the continental United States, where marijuana is banned. In 1982, 6.3 percent of American high school seniors smoked marijuana daily, but only 4 percent did so in Alaska. In 1985, 5.5 percent of American high school seniors used marijuana daily, but in the Netherlands the rate was only 0.5 percent.[4] Those are hardly controlled comparisons—no such comparisons exist—but the numbers that are available do not bear out the drastic scenario portrayed by supporters of continued prohibition.

---

[3]Bureau of the Census, *Historical Statistics of the United States, Colonial Times to 1970* (Washington, 1975), part 1, p. 441.

[4]Arnold Trebach, *The Great Drug War* (New York: Macmillan, 1987), pp. 103, 105.

Figure 1

Combined per Capita Murder and Assault (by Firearm) Rates 1910–43

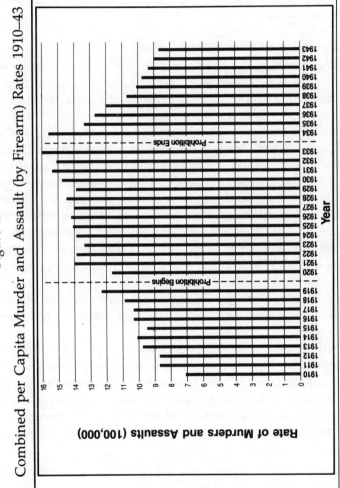

Source: Bureau of the Census, *Historical Statistics of the United States, Colonial Times to 1970* (Washington, 1975), part 1, p. 441.

47

Finally, there is at least some evidence that the "forbidden fruit" aspect of prohibition may lead to increased use of or experimentation with drugs, particularly among the young. That phenomenon apparently occurred with marijuana, LSD, toluene-based glue, and other drugs.[5] The case for legalization does not rely on that argument, but those who believe prohibition needs no defense cannot simply dismiss it.

The Current Crisis of Drug Prohibition

Several recent events have dramatized the failures and costly side effects of the war on drugs: A woman sitting in her kitchen in Washington, D.C., is killed by a stray bullet from a drug dealers' shoot-out. A policeman guarding a witness in a drug case is brutally executed in Queens. In Los Angeles drug-related gang warfare breaks out. General Manuel Noriega engineers a coup d'état in Panama after he is accused of being one of history's great drug dealers. Colombia's courts refuse to extradite major drug dealers to the United States, and its attorney general is brazenly murdered by the Colombian drug cartel. An update of the Kerner Report concludes that the economic status of blacks relative to whites has not improved in 20 years—in part because many blacks are trapped in drug-crime-infested inner cities, where economic progress is slow.

The status quo is intolerable—everyone agrees on that. But there are only two alternatives: further escalate the war on drugs or legalize them.

Escalating the war on drugs is doomed to fail, as it did under President Richard M. Nixon, Gov. Nelson A. Rockefeller, and President Ronald Reagan.[6] It is confronted by a host of seemingly intractable problems: lack of funds, lack of prison space, lack of political will to put middle-class users in jail, and the sheer impossibility of preventing consenting adults in a free society from engaging in

---

[5]See generally, Edward M. Brecher and the editors of Consumers Reports, *Licit and Illicit Drugs* (Boston: Little, Brown, 1972).

[6]On Nixon, see Charles E. Silberman, *Criminal Violence, Criminal Justice* (New York: Vintage Books, 1980), pp. 232–45; on Rockefeller, see National Institute of Law Enforcement and Criminal Justice, *The Nation's Toughest Drug Law: Evaluating the New York Experience*, final report of the Joint Committee on New York Drug Evaluation, March 1978, p. 7; on Reagan, see "The Failure of Enforcement" in this paper.

extremely profitable transactions involving tiny amounts of illegal drugs.

But none of those factors ultimately explains why escalating the war on drugs would fail. Failure is guaranteed because the black market thrives on the war on drugs and benefits from any intensification of it. At best, increased enforcement simply boosts the black-market price of drugs, encouraging more drug suppliers to supply more drugs. The publicized conviction of a drug dealer, by instantly creating a vacancy in the lucrative drug business, has the same effect as hanging up a help-wanted sign saying "Drug dealer needed—$5,000 a week to start—exciting work."

Furthermore, there is a real danger that escalating the war on drugs would squander much of the nation's wealth and freedom, causing enormous social disruption. No limit is yet in sight to the amount of money and new enforcement powers that committed advocates of prohibition will demand before giving up on prohibition.

It is instructive to note the parallel between the current debate over the drug problem and the debate over the alcohol problem in the 1920s and 1930s. In the earlier debate, one side called for intensified enforcement efforts, while the other called for outright repeal. The prohibitionists won all the battles: Enforcement efforts escalated throughout the duration of Prohibition. Convictions rose from 18,000 in 1921 to 61,000 in 1932.[7] Prison terms grew longer and were meted out with greater frequency in the latter years of Prohibition.[8] The enforcement budget rose from $7 million in 1921 to $15 million in 1930—$108 million in 1988 dollars.[9] The number of stills seized rose from 32,000 in 1920 to 282,000 in 1930.[10] In 1926 the Senate Judiciary Committee produced a 1,650-page report evaluating enforcement efforts and proposing reforms.[11] In 1927 the Bureau of Prohibition was created to streamline enforcement efforts, and agents were brought under civil service protection to eliminate corruption and improve professionalism.[12] In 1929 the

[7]*Annual Reports of the Attorney General*, 1921, 1932.

[8]National Commission on Law Observance and Enforcement, *Report on the Enforcement of the Prohibition Laws of the United States*, January 7, 1931, pp. 144–45.

[9]Ibid., p. 18.

[10]Ibid., p. 123; *Annual Report of the Commissioner of Prohibition, 1930*, pp. 110–11.

[11]*Report on the Enforcement*, p. 14.

[12]44 Stats. 1381 (1927).

penalties for violating the National Prohibition Act were increased.[13]

Also in 1929 President Hoover appointed a blue-ribbon commission to evaluate enforcement efforts and recommend reforms. The 1931 Wickersham Commission report (satirized in the poem that serves as the epigraph to this paper), while concluding that "there is as yet no adequate observance or enforcement," nevertheless urged that

> appropriations for the enforcement of the Eighteenth Amendment should be substantially increased and that the vigorous and better organized efforts which have gone on since the Bureau of Prohibition Act, 1927, should be furthered by certain improvements in the statutes and in the organization, personnel, and equipment of enforcement, so as to give enforcement the greatest practical efficiency.[14]

But the proponents of legalization won the war: in 1933, just two years later, Prohibition was dead. In light of this history, it should not be at all surprising that increasing support for drug legalization is coming at the same time that the war on drugs is intensifying.

This paper does not suggest that legalization would solve the drug problem in its entirety. Legalization is offered as a solution only to the "drug-problem problem,"[15] that is, the crime, corruption, and AIDS caused not by the biochemical effects of illegal drugs but by the attempt to fight drug use with the criminal justice system. The repeal of alcohol prohibition provides the appropriate analogy. Repeal did not end alcoholism—as indeed Prohibition did not— but it did solve many of the problems created by Prohibition, such as corruption, murder, and poisoned alcohol. We can expect no more and no less from drug legalization today.

The Burden of Proof

Much of the confusion surrounding drug policy discussions could be alleviated by asking the right question initially. The question that must be addressed in determining whether to legalize drugs is this: do drug laws do more harm than good?

[13]45 Stats. 1446 (1929).

[14]*Report on the Enforcement*, p. 83.

[15]A term coined by Dr. Helen Nowlis. Brecher et al., p. 521.

The focus here is not on how dangerous drugs are or how much damage drug users inflict upon themselves. If those factors were decisive, then surely alcohol and tobacco would be banned. Rather, the proper focus is on how effective drug laws are in preventing damage from drugs compared with the amount of injury the laws themselves cause.

With that emphasis in mind, the respective burdens of proof resting upon the parties to the debate can now be specified. Supporters of prohibition must demonstrate *all* of the following:

(1) that drug use would increase substantially after legalization;

(2) that the harm caused by any increased use would not be offset by the increased safety of legal drug use;

(3) that the harm caused by any increased use would not be offset by a reduction in the use of dangerous drugs that are already legal (e.g., alcohol and tobacco); and

(4) that the harm caused by any increased drug use not offset by (2) or (3) would exceed the harm now caused by the side effects of prohibition (e.g., crime and corruption).

In the absence of data supporting those propositions, neither the theoretical danger of illegal drugs nor their actual harmful effects can be a sufficient basis for prohibition. Neither can the bare fact, if proven, that illegal drug use would rise under legalization.

Prohibitionists face a daunting task—one that no one has yet accomplished or, apparently, even attempted. It might be noted, parenthetically, that a 1984 study by the Research Triangle Institute on the economic costs of drug abuse[16] has been erroneously cited in support of drug prohibition.[17] That report, which estimates the cost of drug abuse at $60 billion for 1983, is not, and was not intended to be, an evaluation of the efficacy of prohibition or the wisdom of legalization. It does not mention the terms "legalization" and "decriminalization" and makes no attempt to separate the costs attributable to drug use per se from the costs attributable to the illegality of drug use. In fact, the study seems to include some costs

---

[16]H. J. Harwood, D. M. Napolitano, P. L. Kristiansen, and J. J. Collins, *Economic Costs to Society of Alcohol and Drug Abuse and Mental Illness* (Research Triangle Park, N.C.: Research Triangle Institute, 1984).

[17]*New York Times*, May 15, 1988, pp. 1, 24; Morton Kondracke, "Don't Legalize Drugs," *New Republic*, June 27, 1988, p. 16; see also, *Time*, May 30, 1988, pp. 14–15.

of *legal* drugs in its estimates.[18] Many of the costs cited are clearly the result of prohibition, for example, interdiction costs ($677 million). Furthermore, the report considers only costs that prohibition has failed to prevent, making no attempt to measure the costs prevented—or caused—by prohibition. In its present form, the study is therefore almost entirely irrelevant to the issue of legalizing drugs.

The case for legalization is sustained if *any* of the following propositions is true:

(1) prohibition has no substantial impact on the level of illegal drug use;

(2) prohibition increases illegal drug use;

(3) prohibition merely redistributes drug use from illegal drugs to harmful legal drugs; or

(4) even though prohibition might decrease the use of illegal drugs, the negative effects of prohibition outweigh the beneficial effects of reduced illegal drug use.

The Costs of Prohibition

As Thomas Sowell writes, "Policies are judged by their consequences, but crusades are judged by how good they make the crusaders feel."[19] So the inquiry must be, do drug laws cause more harm than good?

Street Crime by Drug Users

Drug laws greatly increase the price of illegal drugs, often forcing users to steal to get the money to obtain them. Although difficult to estimate, the black-market prices of heroin and cocaine appear to be about 100 times greater than their pharmaceutical prices. For example, a hospital-dispensed dose of morphine (a drug from which heroin is relatively easily derived) costs only pennies; legal cocaine costs about $20 per ounce. It is frequently estimated that at least 40 percent of all property crimes in the United States are

---

[18]Harwood et al., pp. 49–50.

[19]Thomas Sowell, *Compassion versus Guilt and Other Essays* (New York: William Morrow, 1987), p. 74.

committed by drug users so that they can maintain their habits.[20] That amounts to about 8 million crimes per year and $6 billion in stolen property.[21]

Many studies over a long period have confirmed what every inner-city dweller already knows: drug users steal to get the money to buy expensive illegal drugs. Those studies were reviewed in 1985 in an article entitled "Narcotics and Crime: An Analysis of Existing Evidence for a Causal Relationship." The authors conclude that

> heroin addiction can be shown to dramatically increase property crime levels. . . . A high proportion of addicts' preaddiction criminality consists of minor and drug offenses, while postaddiction criminality is characterized much more by property crime.[22]

Moreover, prohibition also stimulates crime by

● criminalizing users of illegal drugs, which creates disrespect for the law;

● forcing users into daily contact with professional criminals, which often leads to arrest and prison records that make legitimate employment difficult to obtain;

● discouraging legitimate employment because of the need to "hustle" for drug money;

---

[20]Estimates of drug-related crime vary widely. Trebach, summarizing various surveys, puts the figure at 50 percent in urban areas. Arnold Trebach, "The Potential Impact of 'Legal' Heroin in America," in Drugs, Crime, and Politics, ed. Arnold Trebach (New York: Praeger, 1978). A Wharton Econometrics survey found that local police officials believe that drug users commit about 25 percent of auto thefts, 40 percent of robberies and assaults, and 50 percent of burglaries and larcenies. See Gerald G. Godshaw, Hoss K. Koppel, and Russell P. Pancoast, "Anti-Drug Law Enforcement Efforts and Their Impact," prepared for U.S. Customs Service, August 1987. Assistant Police Chief Isaac Fulwood of Washington, D.C., estimated that 50 to 60 percent of crime in his city is drug related. Washington Post, November 7, 1986, p. B1.

[21]Estimate based on victimization surveys done by the Bureau of Justice Statistics for 1985 and the FBI Uniform Crime Reports for 1988, which provide average value of property stolen. Also considered is an unreported crime factor of about 50 percent for less serious crimes, such as larceny. Silberman, pp. 611–13.

[22]George Speckart and M. Douglas Anglin, "Narcotics and Crime: An Analysis of Existing Evidence for a Causal Relationship," Behavioral Sciences and the Law 3 (1985): 273.

- encouraging young people to become criminals by creating an extremely lucrative black market in drugs;
- destroying, through drug crime, the economic viability of low-income neighborhoods, leaving young people fewer alternatives to working in the black market; and
- removing the settling of drug-related disputes from the legal process, which creates a context of violence for the buying and selling of drugs.

Every property crime committed by a drug user is potentially a violent crime. Many victims are beaten and severely injured, and 1,600 are murdered each year.

Black-Market Violence

Prohibition also causes what the media and police misname "drug-related violence." That *prohibition*-related violence includes all the random shootings and murders associated with black-market drug transactions: rip-offs, eliminating the competition, killing informers, and killing suspected informers.

Those who doubt that prohibition is responsible for that violence need only note the absence of violence in the legal drug market. For example, there is no violence associated with the production, distribution, and sale of alcohol. Such violence was ended by the repeal of Prohibition.

The President's Commission on Organized Crime estimates a total of about 70 drug-market murders yearly in Miami alone. Based on that figure and FBI data, a reasonable nationwide estimate would be at least 750 such murders each year.[23] Recent estimates from New York and Washington would suggest an even higher figure.

[23]The base figure is 570, based on an FBI calculation that 3 percent of all murders involved narcotics as the motive. However, that figure is certainly an underestimate since the motive of 25 percent of all murders was "unknown," and drug-related murders can be expected to frequently fall into that category. Testimony in 1984 before the President's Commission on Organized Crime by Dr. Charles V. Welti, deputy chief medical examiner in Miami, indicates that 30 to 40 percent of all murders in Miami—about 70 per year—are drug related. *Record of Hearing IV*, p. 536. One study found that 42 percent of murders in one precinct in New York City were drug related. R. Heffernan, "Homicides Related to Drug Trafficking," *Federal Probation* 3 (September 1982): 3. Those figures indicate that the 3 percent FBI estimate is very low.

About 10 law enforcement officers are killed enforcing drug laws each year. Those people are also victims of drug prohibition.

Do Drugs Cause Crime?

It is often thought that illegal drugs cause crime through their biochemical effects on the mind. In fact, marijuana laws were originally justified on that basis. Today the notion that marijuana causes crime "is no longer taken seriously by even the most ardent [anti-] marijuana propagandists."[24] Regarding heroin:

> There is no doubt that heroin use in and of itself . . . is a neutral act in terms of its potential criminogenic effect upon an individual's behavior. . . .There is nothing in the pharmacology, or physical or psychological impact, of the drug that propels a user to crime.[25]

Cocaine, like other stimulants such as nicotine and caffeine, can stimulate aggressive behavior. However,

> personality and setting as usual make all the difference. . . . Jared Tinkelberg, commenting on a DEA study and in general on the relation between cocaine and violence, expresses some surprise that it seems to produce "amphetamine-like paranoid assaultiveness" so seldom and concludes that at present it is not a serious crime problem. . . . Most violence in the illicit cocaine trade, like the violence in the illicit heroin traffic today and in the alcohol business during Prohibition, is of course not necessarily related to the psychopharmacological properties of the drug. Al Capone did not order murders because he was drunk, and the cocaine dealer "Jimmy" does not threaten his debtors or fear the police because of cocaine-induced paranoia.[26]

When the New York City Police Department announced that 38 percent of murders in the city in 1987 were "drug-related," Deputy Chief Raymond W. Kelly explained:

[24]Erich Goode, *Drugs in American Society*, 2d ed. (New York: Alfred A. Knopf, 1984), p. 124.

[25]Arnold Trebach, *The Heroin Solution* (New Haven, Conn.: Yale University Press, 1982), p. 286.

[26]Lester Grinspoon and James B. Bakalar, *Cocaine—A Drug and Its Social Evolution*, rev. ed. (New York: Basic Books, 1985), p. 227.

When we say drug-related, we're essentially talking about territorial disputes or disputes over possession. . . . We're not talking about where somebody is deranged because they're on a drug. It's very difficult to measure that.[27]

Drugs Made More Dangerous

Because there is no quality control in the black market, prohibition also kills by making drug use more dangerous. Illegal drugs contain poisons, are of uncertain potency, and are injected with dirty needles. Many deaths are caused by infections, accidental overdoses, and poisoning.

At least 3,500 people will die from AIDS each year from using unsterile needles, a greater number than the combined death toll from cocaine and heroin.[28] Those casualties include the sexual partners and children of intravenous drug users. Drug-related AIDS is almost exclusively the result of drug prohibition. Users inject drugs rather than taking them in tablet form because tablets are expensive; they go to "shooting galleries" to avoid arrests for possessing drugs and needles; and they share needles because needles are illegal and thus difficult to obtain. In Hong Kong, where needles are legal, there are *no* cases of drug-related AIDS.[29] Legalization would fight AIDS in three ways:

- by making clean needles cheaply available;
- by making drugs in tablet form less expensive; and
- by helping to break up the drug subculture, with its shooting galleries and needle sharing.

[27]*New York Times*, March 23, 1988, p. B1.

[28]That very conservative estimate is based on the following figures: According to the *AIDS Weekly Surveillance Report*, new cases of drug-related AIDS in 1988 will total more than 6,000. The Centers for Disease Control estimate that 1.5 million Americans carry the AIDS virus and that at least one-fourth of that number will develop the disease itself. Deaths from AIDS in 1991 are expected to total over 50,000. Assuming that the percentage of AIDS cases related to drug use remains about 18 percent, drug-related AIDS deaths would total 9,000 in 1991. According to an unpublished National Institute on Drug Abuse survey, there were 250,000 AIDS-infected drug users in 1987.

[29]*New York Times*, June 17, 1987, p. 1.

As many as 2,400 of the 3,000 deaths attributed to heroin and cocaine use each year—80 percent—are actually caused by black-market factors.[30] For example, many heroin deaths are caused by an allergic reaction to the street mixture of the drug,[31] while 30 percent are caused by infections.[32]

The attempt to protect users from themselves has backfired, as it did during Prohibition. The drug laws have succeeded only in making drug use much more dangerous and in driving it underground, out of the reach of moderating social and medical influences. As indicated in Table 1, drug prohibition causes at least 8,250 deaths each year.[33]

Table 1
Annual Deaths Caused by Drug Prohibition

Cause	Number
Murders incident to street crime	1,600
Black-market murders	750
Drug-related AIDS	3,500
Poisoned drugs/no quality control	2,400
Total	8,250

A point that is implicit throughout this paper should be made explicit here: The users themselves do not benefit from prohibition. Rather, they die of overdoses caused by the uncertain quality of illegal drugs and of AIDS contracted through dirty needles. They are murdered in remarkable numbers while buying or selling drugs. They are led into a criminal lifestyle by the need to raise large sums of money quickly and must associate with professional criminals to

[30]James Ostrowski, "Thinking about Drug Legalization," Cato Institute Policy Analysis no. 121, May 25, 1989, appendix.

[31]Brecher et al., pp. 101–14.

[32]N. Zinberg and J. Robertson, *Drugs and the Public* (New York: Simon & Schuster, 1972), p. 204.

[33]Not included in the estimate are deaths caused by "designer" drugs. Estimates range from 100 to 1,000. "The net effect, tragic and ironic, of drug prohibition has been the creation of synthetic drugs that are more potent, dangerous, and unpredictable than the drugs originally banned. . . . Unless we turn away from drug prohibition, and learn to live with the drugs we have, we will be awash in a flood of cheap and deadly synthetic drug substitutes." Jack Shafer, "The War on Drugs Is Over—The Government Has Lost," *Inquiry*, February 1984, p. 14.

get drugs. Many users have long records of convictions for drug offenses, making it difficult for them to secure legitimate employment. As Randy Barnett notes, "It is difficult to overestimate the harm caused by forcing drug users into a life of crime. Once this threshold is crossed, there is often no return."[34]

And yet, isn't the point of drug prohibition the salvaging of those who, for whatever reasons, are unable to resist the lure of drugs? The 250,000 users infected with AIDS are a grim reminder of the failure of prohibition to do so.[35]

Clogged Courts and Prisons

Each dollar spent enforcing drug laws and fighting the violent crime those laws stimulate is a dollar that cannot be spent fighting other violent crime. The one law enforcement technique that definitely works is the specific deterrence of incarceration. Put a violent career criminal in prison for five years and that person simply will not commit his usual quota of over 100 serious crimes per year.

But right now there are not enough judges and prosecutors to try cases or enough prison spaces to house convicts. In 1987 the federal prison system had 44,000 inmates, including 16,000 drug offenders, while official capacity was only 28,000.[36] About 40 state prison systems are operating under court orders to reduce overcrowding or improve conditions.[37]

Because of the sheer lack of prison space, violent criminals frequently are given deals—probation or shorter terms than they deserve. Then they are back on the streets, and often back to serious crime. For example, in 1987 in New York City, a man who had been released after serving 5 years of a 15-year term for robbery was arrested again for auto theft, released on bail, and finally arrested once more and indicted for rape and robbery at knife point.[38]

[34]Randy E. Barnett, "Curing the Drug-Law Addiction," in *Dealing with Drugs: Consequences of Government Control*, ed. Ronald Hamowy (San Francisco: Pacific Research Institute, 1987), p. 85.

[35]Estimate based on an unpublished study by the National Institute on Drug Abuse. See also "On Drug-Related AIDS and the Legal Ban on Over-the-Counter Hypodermic Needle Sales," report of the Committee on Law Reform of the New York County Lawyers Association, January 12, 1988.

[36]*New York Times*, September 25, 1987.

[37]*New York Times*, March 1, 1987.

[38]*New York Times*, October 23, 1987, p. B5.

In a world of scarce prison resources, sending a drug offender to prison for one year is equivalent to freeing a violent criminal to commit 40 robberies, 7 assaults, 110 burglaries, and 25 auto thefts.[39]

Corruption

Drug money corrupts law enforcement officials. Corruption is a major problem in drug enforcement because drug agents are given tremendous power over desperate persons in possession of large amounts of cash. Drug corruption charges have been leveled against FBI agents, police officers, prison guards, U.S. Customs inspectors, and even prosecutors. In 1986 in New York City's 77th Precinct, 12 police officers were arrested for stealing and selling drugs. Miami's problem is worse. In June 1986 seven officers there were indicted for using their jobs to run a drug operation that used murders, threats, and bribery. Add to that two dozen other cases of corruption in the last three years in Miami alone.

We must question a policy that so frequently turns police officers into organized criminals. Logically, there are two solutions to drug corruption: make police officers morally perfect or eliminate the black market in drugs.

Assault on Civil Liberties

The recent drug hysteria has created an atmosphere in which long-cherished rights are discarded whenever drugs are concerned. Urine testing, roadblocks, routine strip searches, school locker searches without probable cause, preventive detention, and nonjudicial forfeiture of property are now routine weapons in the war on drugs.

Such governmental intrusions into our most personal activities are the natural and necessary consequence of drug prohibition. It is no accident that a law review article entitled "Crackdown: The Emerging 'Drug Exception' to the Bill of Rights" was published in 1987.[40] In explaining why drug prohibition, by its very nature, threatens civil liberties, law professor Randy Barnett notes that drug offenses differ from violent crimes in that there is rarely a

[39]Those figures are based on a 1978 study of the behavior of career criminals. Alfred Blumstein, "Criminal Careers and 'Career Criminals,' " (Washington: National Research Council, 1986).

[40]Steven Wisotsky, "Crackdown: The Emerging 'Drug Exception' to the Bill of Rights," *Hastings Law Journal* 38 (July 1987): 889.

59

complaining witness to a drug transaction.[41] Because drug transactions are illegal but their participants are willing, the transactions are hidden from police view. Thus, to be at all effective, drug agents must intrude into the innermost private lives of *suspected* drug criminals.

The term "innermost" here is no exaggeration. In one case, the Supreme Court "approved a prolonged and humiliating detention of an incomer who was held by customs agents to determine, through her natural bodily processes, whether or not she was carrying narcotics internally," even though probable cause was lacking.[42] In other words, a woman was forced to defecate even though there was no probable cause to believe she was carrying drugs. Because firm evidence of guilt, if it exists, is not obtained until *after* such intrusions, the privacy of large numbers of innocent people must be violated in the process of enforcing drug laws.

The same principle operates in enforcement efforts seemingly far removed from the invasive practice of body searches. Roadblocks, used with greater frequency in the war on drugs, impose an inconvenience on all citizens for the sake of allowing the police to ferret out a few drug suspects. One of the main purposes of currency reporting laws is to allow government agents to trace cash from drug transactions that is being "laundered." Currently, most cash transactions involving more than $10,000 must be reported to the government. Thus, to allow government agents to search for a relatively small number of drug criminals, the financial privacy of *all* must be sacrificed. That intrusion is simply another cost of criminalizing an activity in which all the participants are willing.

The dangerous precedents described here are tolerated in the war on drugs, but they represent a permanent increase in government power for all purposes. The tragedy is how cheaply our rights have been sold. Our society was once one in which the very thought of men and women being strip searched and forced to urinate in the presence of witnesses was revolting. That now seems like a long time ago. And all this for a policy that simply does not work, since it is prohibition itself that causes the very problems that make extreme measures seem necessary to a befuddled public.

[41]Barnett, in Hamowy, pp. 88–89.

[42]*People* v. *Luna*, 1989 WL 13231 (N.Y. Court of Appeals, 1989) discussing *U.S.* v. *de Hernandez*, 473 U.S. 531 (1985).

Destruction of Community

Drug prohibition has had devastating effects on inner-city minority communities. A poorly educated young person in the inner city now has three choices: welfare, a low-wage job, or the glamorous and high-profit drug business. It is no wonder that large numbers of ghetto youth have gone into drug dealing, some of them as young as 10 years old. When the most successful people in a community are those engaged in illegal activities, the natural order of the community is destroyed. A *New York Times* article reported that "the underground drug economy . . . puts more power in the hands of teen-agers" and makes the entire community more violent.[43] How can a mother maintain authority over a 16-year-old son who pays the rent out of his petty cash? How can a teacher persuade students to study hard when dropouts drive BMWs? The profits from prohibition make a mockery of the work ethic and of family authority.

A related problem is that prohibition also forces drug users to come into contact with people of real criminal intent. For all the harm that alcohol and tobacco do, one does not have to deal with criminals to use those drugs. Prohibition drags the drug user into a criminal culture.

Once used to breaking the law by using drugs and to dealing with criminals, it is hard for the drug user and especially the drug dealer to maintain respect for other laws. Honesty, respect for private property, and other marks of a law-abiding community are further casualties of the drug laws. When the huge illegal profits and violence of the illegal drug business permeate a neighborhood, it ceases to be a functioning community. The consequences range from discouragement of legitimate businesses, to disdain for education, to violence that makes mail carriers and ambulance drivers afraid to enter housing complexes. The destruction of inner-city communities must be judged one of the major evils of prohibition.

The Consequences of Legalization

As a general rule, legal drug use is less dangerous than illegal drug use and is influenced by the mores of society. Legal drug use

---

[43]Gina Kolata, "Grim Seeds of Park Rampage Found in East Harlem Streets," *New York Times*, May 2, 1989.

involves nonlethal doses, nonpoisoned drugs, clean needles, and warning labels. The night basketball star Len Bias died from a cocaine overdose, his friends, fearing the police, waited until after his third seizure before calling an ambulance. Illegal drug users have been arrested at hospitals after seeking medical attention. Legalization would put an end to that kind of nonsense. Users would be free to seek medical attention or counseling, if needed, and would not be alienated from family and friends as many are now. For a drug user to kill himself with drugs under those conditions would be tantamount to suicide.

A given amount of legal drug use would cause much less death and illness than the same amount of illegal drug use. A realistic estimate is that illegal drug use is five times more dangerous than legal use.[44] Thus, even a highly unlikely fivefold increase in drug use under legalization would *not* increase the current number of drug overdose deaths. The yearly number of heroin and cocaine deaths combined is about 3,000. Eighty percent, or 2,400, are caused by black-market factors; 20 percent, or 600, are caused by the intrinsic effects of the drugs. If, under legalization, legal use remained at the same level as current illegal use, there would be only 600 deaths each year. Only a 500 percent increase in use would match the current black-market death toll. (Note that historians' estimates of the increase in alcohol use in the decades after the repeal of Prohibition range from zero to a maximum of 250 percent.[45])

Furthermore, it would take a 1,275 percent increase in legal drug use to produce as many deaths as drug prohibition—through murder, AIDS, and poisoned drugs—is already causing. Prohibition now causes 8,250 deaths, while 600 are the result of the drugs themselves. Thus, for legalized drug use to match the overall death toll of prohibition, use would have to increase more than 13-fold.

There are now about 5 million regular cocaine users and 500,000 regular heroin users. To prove that prohibition saves more lives than it destroys, one would have to show that legalization would result in more than 6.5 million *additional* heroin users and more than 65 million *additional* cocaine users. Such enormous increases

[44]Ostrowski, appendix.

[45]See Kyvig, pp. 24, 112–113, 131, 186; Robert O'Brien and Morris Chafetz, *Encyclopedia of Alcoholism* (New York: Facts on File Publications, 1982), pp. 72–73; Kondracke, p. 17.

are inconceivable at a time when the overall trend is toward *less* legal and illegal drug use.

Drug Switching

However, even if prohibition advocates could prove that such astronomical increases would occur, prohibition would still not be vindicated because of "drug switching."

Any increase in the use of newly legalized drugs is likely to involve some drug switching by smokers and drinkers. Since the death rate for those activities is greater than the death rate for heroin, cocaine, and marijuana, any deaths avoided by switching would have to be subtracted from the deaths caused by the legal use of heroin and cocaine. (The marijuana death rate is apparently zero.) Depending on the rate of switching, it is possible that the increased use of those drugs could actually reduce the total number of drug deaths.

For example, assume that legalization led to 10 million new cocaine users, which, all else being equal, could cause an additional 400 deaths per year. However, assume also that a mere 5 percent of those users switched to cocaine from tobacco (tobacco and cocaine both stimulate the central nervous system). Tobacco-related deaths would eventually decrease by about 3,250 per year, and the result would be a net gain in lives saved of 2,850.[46]

Drug switching is a critical issue that any regime of drug control must face. What is the point of attempting to limit access to certain drugs when the user merely turns to other, more dangerous drugs? For example, opium use in China may or may not have been vastly reduced, but "weak tranquilizers and sedative pills have been widely used in China, and they are easily available on the market."[47] Furthermore, two-thirds of all Chinese men now smoke cigarettes.[48]

[46]Using the more sophisticated method of "years of potential life lost" would be unlikely to change the analysis significantly. Although people who die from alcohol and tobacco use are generally older than those who die from illegal drug use, alcohol and tobacco also cause a significant number of sudden deaths that take the lives of people of all ages (e.g., car accidents, fires).

[47]Chinese journalist Shen Chenru claims that the Communist Chinese government completely eliminated the opium problem three years after coming to power and that "drug-taking became extinct." But in the same article, he admits that heroin is being smuggled into China and that 18 people were charged with drug trafficking in one month in a city there. Shen Chenru, "Keeping Narcotics under Strict Control: Some Effects in China," *Impact of Science on Society* 34, no. 1 (1984): 136.

[48]CBS News, April 24, 1988.

Examples of drug switching abound. When narcotics were first outlawed, many middle-class users switched to "barbiturates . . . and later, to sedatives and tranquilizers. . . . The laws did nothing to terminate this group of addicts. . . . They simply changed the drug to which the users were addicted."[49] Marijuana smoking first became popular as a replacement for alcohol during Prohibition. Similarly, it is common for alcoholics trying to stay sober to take up tobacco smoking instead. Recently, it has been reported that some intravenous heroin users have switched to smoking crack to avoid the risk of AIDS.

In sum, even if prohibitionists can prove that the use of drugs would greatly increase under legalization and that the increase would not be offset by gains in drug quality, they must then show that new users would not be switching from more dangerous drugs (e.g., alcohol) to less dangerous drugs (e.g., opium). They must also prove that the damage caused by any increase in legal use would exceed the tremendous damage, both social and medical, caused by the current level of illegal use. Until those proofs are given, prohibition will remain a policy in search of a justification.

Would Drug Use Increase?

Long-term trends in legal drug use suggest that there would be no substantial increase in drug use under decriminalization. As a society, we are gradually moving away from the harmful use of alcohol and tobacco:

> In 1956, 42 percent of adults smoked; in 1980, only 33 percent. In 1977, 29 percent of high school seniors smoked; in 1981, 20 percent. . . . We did not declare a war on tobacco. We did not make it illegal. . . . We did seek to convince our citizens not to smoke through persuasion, objective information, and education.[50]

Alcohol consumption and deaths caused by alcohol have also been gradually declining as people switch from hard liquor to less potent

[49]Goode, p. 221.

[50]Arnold Trebach, "Peace without Surrender in the Perpetual Drug War," *Justice Quarterly* 1 (1984): 136.

formulations.[51] Finally, use of marijuana—now a de facto legal drug in many states—declined 11 percent from 1982 to 1985, according to the National Institute on Drug Abuse.

As our society grows increasingly health and fitness conscious, heavy drug use loses its appeal. Many people are trading the tavern for the health club and choosing vitamins instead of martinis. The values of health and moderation clearly have less influence on the illegal drug scene, where hard-core drug users form subcultures that reinforce heavy, reckless drug use.

It is a mistake to assume that the mere availability of a drug leads to its use or abuse:

> For most of human history, even under conditions of ready access to the most potent of drugs, people and societies have regulated their drug use without requiring massive education, legal, and interdiction campaigns.[52]

In both America and England, narcotics use peaked and then declined long before national prohibition was adopted.[53] Today, in spite of the availability of alcohol, problem drinkers are thought to compose only about 10 percent of the population.[54] In spite of the fact that marijuana can be purchased on virtually any street corner in some cities, only about 10 percent of the population has done so in the last month, according to NIDA. Significantly, the figures for cocaine are quite similar, in spite of the drug's reputation for addictiveness. About 20 million people have tried the drug, but only 25 percent of that number have used it in the last month and only about 10 percent are considered addicts.[55] It bears remembering that for cocaine, the sample population is drawn from that

[51]Per capita alcohol consumption declined 0.7 percent from 1974 to 1984, while distilled spirit consumption declined 15.4 percent. Total deaths caused directly by alcohol declined 12 percent over the period even as the population rose. *Morbidity and Mortality Weekly Report* 35, no. 2SS, Centers for Disease Control, August 1986.

[52]Stanton Peele, "A Moral Vision of Addiction: How People's Values Determine Whether They Become and Remain Addicts," *Journal of Drug Issues* 17 (Spring 1987): 209.

[53]David F. Musto, "The History of Legislative Control over Opium, Cocaine, and Their Derivatives," in Hamowy, pp. 41–42.

[54]Brecher et al., p. 260.

[55]Testimony of Dr. Arnold Washton before the President's Commission on Organized Crime, November 27, 1984. *Record of Hearing IV*, p. 11.

segment of the population already interested enough in drugs to break the law to obtain them. Thus, an even lower percentage of repeat users could be expected from the overall population under legalization. Those numbers support Stanton Peele's belief that "cocaine use is now described [incorrectly] as presenting the same kind of lurid monomania that pharmacologists once claimed only heroin could produce."[56]

The fatal flaw in the policy of prohibition is that those who need to be protected most from drug use—hard-core users—are at the same time those least likely to be deterred by laws against drugs. For those individuals, drug use is one of the highest values in life. They will take great risks, pay high prices, and violate the law in pursuit of that value.

Further, it is naive to think that prohibition relieves prospective or even moderate drug users of the need to make responsible decisions with respect to illegal drugs. It is just too easy and inexpensive to obtain a few batches of crack or heroin to claim that prohibition obviates individual choice. Individual preference—not law enforcement—is the likely explanation for the existence of 20 million marijuana smokers but only 500,000 heroin users. If 20 million people demanded heroin, the black market would meet that demand, perhaps with synthetic substitutes, just as it met the enormous demand for alcohol in the 1920s. Prohibition is at best a comforting illusion.

Perhaps the most telling indicator of the ineffectiveness of U.S. drug laws is their failure to reduce the overall use of illegal drugs. On a per capita basis, the use of narcotics was no more prevalent before prohibition than it is today, and the use of cocaine is more widespread today than when it was legally available. In 1915, the year the first national control laws became effective, there were about 200,000 regular narcotics users and only 20,000 regular cocaine users.[57] Today there are about 500,000 regular heroin users and 2 million regular cocaine users.[58] (Opium and morphine, also

[56]Peele, p. 200.

[57]Lawrence Kolb and A. G. Du Mez, "The Prevalence and Trend of Drug Addiction in the United States and the Factors Influencing It," U.S. Public Health Reports 39 (May 23, 1924): 1179ff.

[58]Numbers based on an unpublished study by the National Institute on Drug Abuse.

66

narcotics, have essentially been driven out of circulation by the more profitable heroin. Prohibition has not reduced narcotics use, but it has made narcotics more powerful.) Thus, with a population more than twice what it was in 1915, the percentage of the population using narcotics has remained about the same, while cocaine use has increased by more than 4,000 percent. Seventy years of intensive law enforcement efforts have failed to measurably reduce drug use.

The failure of drug control should not be surprising. During Prohibition, alcohol consumers merely switched from beer and wine to hard liquor, often of dubious quality, resulting in a drastic increase in deaths from alcohol poisoning.[59] Whether Prohibition actually reduced total consumption is disputed,[60] but it is known that the repeal of Prohibition did not lead to an explosive increase in drinking.[61] More recently, in those states that have decriminalized marijuana, no substantial increase in use has occurred.[62] When the Netherlands decriminalized marijuana in 1978, use actually declined.[63]

The Failure of Enforcement

Common sense indicates that illegal drugs will always be readily available. Prison wardens cannot keep drugs out of their own institutions—an important lesson for those who would turn this country into a prison to stop drug use. Police officers are regularly caught using drugs, selling drugs, *stealing* drugs. How are those people going to lead a drug war?

[59]Sean Cashman, *Prohibition—The Lie of the Land* (New York: Macmillan, 1981), pp. 251–56.

[60]Kyvig, pp. 24, 112–13.

[61]Ibid., p. 186. Some commentators have cited the sizable alcohol consumption rates in postwar America as evidence that Prohibition repeal may have been unwise. But surely some of the increase in consumption was due to the increased purchasing power of Americans in that era and not solely to the legal availability of alcohol. It is reasonable to assume that even if Prohibition had not been repealed, an increase in disposable income would have led to increased alcohol consumption.

[62]"Monitoring the Future: A Continuing Study of Lifestyles and Values of Youth," (Ann Arbor, Mich.: National Institute on Drug Abuse, University of Michigan, 1986).

[63]Kevin Zeese, "No More Drug War," *National Law Journal* (July 7, 1986): 32, citing Scientific Study of Alcohol and Drug Use, "The Use of Drugs, Alcohol, and Tobacco," Netherlands Ministry of Welfare, Health, and Cultural Affairs, 1985.

Regarding the Reagan administration's enforcement efforts, the *New York Times* reported on September 4, 1986:

> Four and a half years after Vice President Bush established the South Florida Task Force, the most ambitious and expensive drug enforcement operation in the nation's history, the Federal officials who run it say they have barely dented the drug trade here.

On August 10, 1986, a *Times* analysis concluded that "20 years of intensive enforcement has done little to reduce drug abuse." The same article quoted Judge Irving R. Kaufman: "Law enforcement has been tested to the utmost, but let's face it, it just hasn't worked." And even President Reagan admitted that "all the confiscation and law enforcement in the world will not cure this plague." Law enforcement die-hards should take note of the failure of the death penalty—liberally applied—to stop drugs in Malaysia. Despite 18 death sentences and 4 executions, "authorities reported the widespread use of illicit drugs."[64]

A 1988 General Accounting Office report recently released at the White House Conference for a Drug-Free America contains overwhelming evidence of the failure of the Reagan administration's war on drugs.[65] Contrary to the claims of some critics, the war on drugs did not fail for lack of effort. The federal drug control budget increased from $1.2 billion in 1981 to nearly $4 billion in 1987. The FBI and the military were brought into drug enforcement. Two major pieces of legislation were passed to toughen penalties and give enforcers more powers: the Comprehensive Crime Control Act of 1984 and the Anti-Drug Abuse Act of 1986. Arrests rose 58 percent and federal prisons became filled with convicted drug dealers. Drug seizures greatly increased—362 percent in the case of cocaine. The GAO reported the results:

- "Drug abuse in the United States has persisted at a very high level throughout the 1980s."
- *Cocaine*. The amount of cocaine consumed more than doubled. The price declined about 30 percent. The average purity doubled. Cocaine-related deaths rose substantially.

[64]Arnold Trebach, "The Lesson of Ayatollah Khalkali," *Journal of Drug Issues* (Fall 1981): 383–84.
[65]General Accounting Office, *Controlling Drug Abuse: A Status Report, 1988.*

- *Heroin.* The price of heroin declined 20 percent. The average purity rose 33 percent. Heroin-related deaths rose substantially.
- *Marijuana.* While use has declined, "marijuana continues to be readily available in most areas of the country, with a trend toward increased potency levels." Marijuana is now grown in all 50 states and "to avoid detection, marijuana growers are moving their operations indoors and are growing smaller and more scattered plots outdoors."

In short, prohibition has failed to eliminate or even seriously reduce the use of illegal drugs.

Why Prohibition Fails

The reasons for the failure of wars on drugs are best seen by examining the motivations of drug users, sellers, and enforcers.

Drugs have a direct, powerful effect on human consciousness and emotions. Drug laws, on the other hand, have only an occasional impact on the drug user. For the many users who continue to take drugs even after being penalized by law, the subjective benefits of drugs outweigh the costs of criminal penalties.

Even where there are not criminal sanctions, many users continue to take drugs despite the severe physical penalties drugs impose on their bodies. Again, they simply consider the psychic benefit of drug use more important than the physical harm. The fact is, drugs motivate some people—those who most need protection from them—more than any set of penalties a civilized society can impose, and even more than those that some less-than-civilized societies have imposed. The undeniable seductiveness of drugs, usually considered a justification for prohibition, thus actually argues for legalization. The law simply cannot deter millions of people deeply attracted to drugs; it can only greatly increase the social costs of drug use.

As for drug sellers, they are simply more highly motivated than those who are paid to stop them. Drug sellers make enormous profits—much more than they could make at legal jobs—and they are willing to risk death and long prison terms to do so. They are professionals, are on the job 24 hours a day, and are able to pour huge amounts of capital into their enterprises. They are willing to murder competitors, informers, and police as needed.

On the other hand, law enforcement officers get paid whether they catch drug dealers or not. They have virtually no economic stake in the success of their efforts, aside from incremental salary increases. While it is true that police officers also risk their lives in their jobs, drug dealers face a much greater risk of violent death— perhaps 100 times greater. Drug dealers have 10 times as much money to work with as do drug enforcers. Drug enforcement is a bureaucracy and suffers from all the inefficiencies of bureaucracies,[66] while drug dealers are entrepreneurs, unrestrained by arbitrary bureaucratic rules and procedures. They do what needs to be done according to their own judgment and, unlike drug enforcers, are not restrained by the law.

The public has the false impression that drug enforcers are highly innovative, continually devising new schemes to catch drug dealers. Actually, the reverse is true. The dealers, like successful businessmen, are usually one step ahead of the "competition":

> Private firms [read: drug dealers] are constantly seeking new products and practices to give them a competitive edge. They adapt swiftly to changing market conditions, knowing that the failure to do so might lead to bankruptcy.
>
> The rate of innovation in public operations [DEA] is much slower, and public services [drug enforcement] appear to change very slowly over time. During the time when a private-sector good or service may change beyond recognition, the public sector seems to turn out the same products year after year. The low rate of innovation in the state's postal services, for example, contrasts sharply with innovations of private postal services.[67]

Finally, drug dealers can use their enormous profits to bribe the police. A minority of enforcement agents will always decide that the monetary benefit of a bribe is more important than the moral cost and legal risk, particularly when it is so clear that their legitimate enforcement efforts have been futile. Drugs are available in prisons not because friends and relatives smuggle them in but because corrupt prison guards are eager to supplement their income.

[66]Those inefficiencies are detailed by Madsen Pirie in *Dismantling the State: The Theory and Practice of Privatization* (Dallas: National Center for Policy Analysis, 1985).
[67]Ibid., pp. 12–13.

It is easy to get lost in piles of numbers, names, dates, and places when evaluating the effect of drug enforcement. But it is more important to keep in mind the ultimately decisive facts of human motivation. Those facts guarantee that wars on drugs will always fail.

The Policy Alternatives

Reform alternatives to prohibition can best be seen as gradations leading from outright criminal prohibition to outright free availability. The main options are presented in Table 2.

Table 2

Alternatives to Prohibition

Option	Description
Status quo: prohibition	Criminal ban on production, sale, and use
Option A: decriminalization (new British system)	Government-controlled distribution through clinics only for short-term treatment; criminal penalties for unauthorized sale and use
Option B: decriminalization	Government-controlled distribution through clinics for long-term maintenance; criminal penalties for unauthorized sale and use
Option C: decriminalization (old British system)	Government-controlled distribution; availability by prescription from any physician for treatment or maintenance; criminal penalties for nonprescription sale and use
Option D: legalization (British and American systems before 1914)	Distribution, sale, and use regulated on a par with the alcoholic beverage industry; nonprescription use by adults permitted

The arguments presented earlier indicate that Option D, legalization, would be the best choice. Nonprescription availability was public policy in the United States and England with respect to narcotics until 1914 and is still public policy today with respect to alcohol and tobacco. As noted, the medical dangers of alcohol and tobacco are even greater than those of heroin or cocaine. There is simply no logical basis for the different legal treatment of those drugs. When prohibitionists attempting to articulate a distinguishing criterion confront the clear evidence of tobacco's and alcohol's greater deadliness, they lamely assert that the distinction is simply that legislatures have chosen to treat them differently. This is question begging in its purest form: the very issue in dispute is the rationality of that choice.

In its simplest terms, the choice between decriminalization and legalization is a choice between solving part of the problem and solving the entire problem, or close to it. Since the black market in illegal drugs is the cause of most drug-related problems, the goal of reform should be to *eliminate the black market.* Legalization would do that; decriminalization would not. For example, dispensing drugs in federal clinics staffed by psychiatrists would probably draw some business away from the black market. But users who did not want to be treated by psychiatrists or take drugs in a clinical setting would continue to fuel a violent and destructive black market. How many drinkers would go to a hospital to drink liquor while being harangued by psychiatrists?

The British Systems, Old and New

Since the goal of reform is to eliminate the black market and its attendant problems, the only valid test for judging the success or failure of reform is whether that goal has been accomplished. However, opponents of decriminalization or legalization sometimes proffer different criteria for evaluating the results of reform. The prime example is embodied in their ubiquitous claim that "the British system failed"; they point to the fact that overall heroin use in England rose substantially during the 1960s, when doctors were allowed to prescribe heroin on a long-term basis. However, their evaluation of the old British system cannot withstand scrutiny.

In the 1920s the British elected to follow the "medical model" of drug control (while the United States adopted the "criminal model"). Private physicians were allowed discretion in prescribing heroin and other controlled drugs for their patients. By most accounts, the system worked fairly well for the next 40 years: the number of users remained low, they received quality-controlled drugs under medical supervision, and no substantial black market developed.

However, in the 1960s heroin use increased substantially, especially among the young. The new users received heroin from illegal imports and from "gray market" sellers, users who received large amounts of prescribed heroin from a few cooperative physicians.

In response to that situation, the system was altered in the late 1960s. The right of individual physicians to prescribe heroin was revoked, and Drug Treatment Centers were set up to treat users. While heroin could still be prescribed at DTCs, the emphasis shifted to "curing" users instead of maintaining them on a long-term basis. As a result, prescription of heroin in England today as slowed to a trickle.

To argue that the system *caused* the increased use of heroin in England in the 1960s is to confuse correlation with causation. If the system caused increased drug use in the 1960s, why did it not do the same during the preceding four decades it was in effect? And if the system caused increased use in Britain, what caused the similar increase in the United States during the same period? It should be noted that drug use in England continued to rise even under the new British system.

Neither the American nor the British systems—nor any other system—have been able to stop intermittent increases in drug use. As Arnold Trebach writes:

> The clinics . . . were instructed to stop the spread of heroin addiction in the general population. But no one—not the second Brain committee, not the other experienced drug abuse doctors, not the criminologists, not the police, and certainly not the visiting American experts—knew then, and no one knows now, how to perform that task.[68]

Erich Goode concurs:

> There is at present no possible solution to the drug problem. There is no program in effect or under discussion that offers any hope whatsoever of a "solution." Asking for the solution to the drug problem is a little like asking for the solution

[68]Trebach, *The Heroin Solution*, p. 220.

to the accident problem, the problem of crime and violence, the problems created by the economy.[69]

Given that neither the old British nor the American system stopped drug use, which minimized the social harmfulness of drug use? The obvious answer is the old British system, under which there was virtually no black market or organized crime and little drug-related crime or violence. Users were better off too, since they received quality-controlled drugs and medical treatment and were not branded as criminals and social outcasts.

When the British moved toward the criminal model of drug control, the effective termination of heroin maintenance forced users to turn to the black market, leading to an "explosion of heroin importation"[70] in the 1980s:

> The evidence suggests that the illicit market in heroin, and the involvement of criminal syndicates, increased in direct relationship to the policy of the clinics in rapidly cutting heroin prescribing.[71]

Arnold Trebach agrees:

> Inspector [H.B.] Spear is convinced that the new crop of younger addicts, having been repelled in various ways by the clinics, is resorting to the street, to the black market, and to crime in order to obtain money to buy drugs. . . . Detective Chief Inspector Colin Coxall estimated in July 1979 that 3,700 heroin addicts were on the streets of London using illegal drugs and that these addicts were spending between 60 and 80 pounds per day to support their habits. Most were forced to resort to crime in order to find that much money. He calculated that 147 million pounds (approximately $382 million) worth of illegal heroin was being traded on the streets of London annually.[72]

Even the British government now acknowledges a "growing incidence of serious crime associated with the illegal supply of controlled drugs" and describes the drug problem as "the most serious

[69]Goode, p. 253.
[70]Editorial, *British Journal of Addiction* 82 (1987): 457.
[71]Kenneth Leach, "Leaving It to the Market," *New Statesman*, January 4, 1985, p. 9.
[72]Trebach, *The Heroin Solution*, p. 212.

peacetime threat to our national well-being."[73] By adopting the American criminal model of drug control, the British created an American-style drug problem within only a few years.

Since the black market in illegal drugs is the source of most drug-related problems, that market must be eliminated to the greatest extent possible. The most efficient means of doing so is legalization.

Hope for the Future

It is clear that most of the serious problems the public associates with illegal drug use are, in reality, caused directly or indirectly by drug prohibition.

Let's assume the war on drugs is given up as the misguided enterprise it is. What will happen? The day after legalization goes into effect, the streets of America will be safer. The drug dealers will be gone. The shoot-outs between drug dealers will end. Innocent bystanders will not be murdered anymore. Hundreds of thousands of drug "addicts" will no longer roam the streets, shoplifting, mugging, breaking into homes in the middle of the night to steal, and dealing violently with those who happen to wake up. One year after prohibition is repealed, 1,600 innocent people who would otherwise have been dead at the hands of drug criminals will be alive.

Within days of prohibition repeal, thousands of judges, prosecutors, and police will be free to catch, try, and imprison violent career criminals—criminals who commit 50 to 100 serious crimes, including robbery, rape, and murder, per year when on the loose. For the first time in years, our overcrowded prisons will have room for them. Ultimately, repeal of prohibition will open 75,000 jail cells.

The day after repeal, organized crime will get a big pay cut—$80 billion a year.

How about those slick young drug dealers who are the new role models for the youth of the inner cities, with their designer clothes and Mercedes convertibles, always wearing a broad, smug smile that says crime pays? They snicker at the honest kids going to school or to work at the minimum wage. The day after repeal, the honest kids will have the last laugh. The dealers will be out of a job, unemployed.

[73]British Information Services, "The Prevention and Treatment of Drug Misuse in Britain," 1985, p. 1.

The day after repeal, real drug education can begin and, for the first time in history, it can be honest. No more need to prop up the failed war on drugs.

The year before repeal, 500,000 Americans will have died from illnesses related to overeating and lack of exercise,[74] 390,000 from smoking, and 150,000 from drinking alcohol. About 3,000 will have died from cocaine, heroin, and marijuana combined, with many of those deaths the result of the lack of quality control in the black market. The day after repeal, cocaine, heroin, and marijuana will, by and large, do no harm to those who choose not to consume them. In contrast, the day before prohibition repeal, all Americans, whether or not they choose to use illegal drugs, will be forced to endure the violence, street crime, erosion of civil liberties, corruption, and social and economic decay caused by the war on drugs.

That is why drug legalization unavoidably becomes a moral issue. The war on drugs is immoral as well as impractical. It imposes enormous costs, including the ultimate cost of death, on large numbers of non-drug-abusing citizens in the failed attempt to save a relatively small group of hard-core drug abusers from themselves. It is immoral and absurd to *force* some people to bear costs so that others may be prevented from *choosing* to do harm to themselves. This crude utilitarian sacrifice—so at odds with traditional American values—has never been, and can never be, justified. That is why the war on drugs must be ended and why it *will* be ended once the public comes to understand the truth about our present destructive policy.

[74]One million Americans die each year from cardiovascular diseases. According to Dr. Regan Bradford of the National Heart, Lung, and Blood Institute, in countries with lower fat diets, such as Japan, the cardiovascular death rate is only about one-tenth the U.S. rate (personal communication, June 21, 1988).

How to Win the War on Drugs

Charles Murray

There's something unpleasantly familiar about the debate over
the War on Drugs: It bears a strong resemblance to the debate over
the war in Vietnam. The sides are divided into hawks who tell us
the war is winnable if we just send in a few more divisions, and
doves—the legalizers—who think the war shouldn't be fought. The
hawks don't want to talk about how much victory will really cost,
and the doves don't want to talk about the consequences if their
scenarios about the post-surrender future are wrong. Each side
includes many who favor their solution less because it promises to
work than because of their world view—one that may or may not
be relevant. Could it be that we need a different way of looking at
the drug problem that yields a different set of solutions?

Let me begin by putting my own biases on the table. In principle,
I am a dove. If someone who is high on drugs goes out and robs,
rapes, or pillages, he should have the book thrown at him; but it
does not follow that the act of taking a drug is in itself something
that the government needs to prohibit. I am not persuaded by the
Tories who want to use the instruments of the federal government
to promote virtue. Nor do I worry about the potential costs of
legalization, because I don't accept that drug users who find themselves unable to function have thereby earned a legal claim on their
fellow citizens' support.

That being said, I cannot bring myself to support a federal law
legalizing drugs right now, as a single, isolated change in social
policy. For though I am confident that legalization would work in
a society where people are held responsible for the consequences
of their actions, that's not the way contemporary America works.
In the same inner-city areas where the drug problem is worst, I can

Charles Murray is Bradley Fellow at the Manhattan Institute and the author of *In
Pursuit: Of Happiness and Good Government*.
This article is reprinted, with permission, from The *New Republic*, May 21, 1990.

too easily neglect my children without being called to account, fail to hold a job and still have food to eat and a place to live, or be a vicious nuisance to my neighbors with impunity. These kinds of behavior, which drug addiction often induces, must be subject to social and economic sanctions if legalization is to work. To legalize drugs in America as of 1990 is to give people the right to be responsible for themselves without also obliging them to do so. It is a dangerous mix. Furthermore, I'm a father, and maybe keeping drugs illegal makes it easier for me to keep my children off drugs. On the drug issue, I'm a libertarian who has been willing to sell out.

The War on Drugs has made that compromise much harder to live with. The analogy with Vietnam is again apt: The hawks still like to talk about body counts—the number of pounds of cocaine seized, flashy convictions—instead of telling us what ground has been taken and held. The hawks' arguments are still larded with invective—once again, the doves must be cowards. What the public needs to see is some specific, hard-headed analysis of how we can win this war at an affordable price. And that is what the hawks fail to explain.

The *National Drug Control Strategy* produced by William Bennett's office is a case in point. The *Strategy* is written by people who have done their homework—and it is quite modest in the claims it makes about our experience with interdiction, rehabilitation, education, and law enforcement. Then comes the appendix, presenting its quantified two- and ten-year objectives. The ten-year objectives call for 50 percent reductions in a wide variety of important indicators of drug use—an ambitious set of goals indeed. But the goals have no link with the discussion that preceded them.

Interdiction offers a good example. The depressing facts have been well publicized. In 1975 the U.S. Customs Service seized just 729 pounds of cocaine during the entire year, and the price of a pure gram (in 1987 dollars) was $1,200. In 1987 it seized forty-four *tons* of cocaine, and the price of a pure gram was $143, roughly one-ninth of the price twelve years earlier. From 1986 to 1987 Customs' cocaine seizures increased by a prodigious eighteen tons—after which the typical gram of cocaine on the street was purer than it had been a year earlier and still cost the same.

The authors of the *Strategy* obviously had contemplated these figures, and nowhere in the text did the authors claim that increased interdiction efforts would reduce supply on the street. And yet the ten-year objective for the War on Drugs as stated in the appendix is "a 50 percent reduction in estimated amounts of cocaine, marijuana, heroin, and dangerous drugs entering the United States." How? Is the goal of a 50 percent reduction just window dressing, complying with a congressional requirement to devise quantified goals? If so, someone should admit that, and then tell us what a reasonable expectation might be. Going by the record so far, the billions being spent on interdiction is money down the drain.

An even more troubling example of the inconsistency between experience and rhetoric in the War on Drugs involves law enforcement. The Strategy argues (correctly, I think) that law enforcement has gotten an unfairly bad rap. A substantial body of evidence confirms that enforcement can raise the monetary costs, the search costs, and the risks of punishment involved in using drugs, and thus discourage drug use. The difficulty lies in trying to apply this evidence to the contemporary drug problem. The only large-scale success in drug control that has been claimed involves the stabilization of the heroin user population in the early 1970s, as described recently by James Q. Wilson in an influential article in Commentary. I think Wilson is too quick to credit the effect to drug policy—this was the period when cocaine was the chic new drug among the same urban black population that had formerly used heroin. But even accepting Wilson's account, the chief mechanisms for affecting the heroin trade are said to have been a temporary disruption of supply from Turkey and an increased fear of the health risks. The only evidence that raising the criminal risks for small-time dealers and users works is based on small, highly targeted, extremely resource-intensive efforts, in which success lasts for only a few months after the cleanup ends. This doesn't invalidate the theory. Apply the same pressure everywhere, and maybe we would suppress drug use everywhere. But this is where the gap between the conceivable and the possible becomes an abyss.

The Impossibility of Deterrence

A simple exercise will illustrate the nature of the problem. We begin by stipulating that deterrence works if risk is raised sufficiently, and then contemplate the implications of raising that risk. Then we try to plug in some numbers.

According to the 1988 version of the government-sponsored annual survey, 28 million persons used an illicit drug within that year. According to the FBI's figures, there were 839,000 arrests for possession of drugs that year—less than 3 percent of all users after taking multiple arrests of the same person into account. In that same year 317,000 persons were arrested for trafficking or manufacture. No one knows what percentage of all dealers this represents. Now fill in the blanks: What percentage of users and how many dealers must we arrest and meaningfully punish to achieve a major reduction in drug use? I am willing to entertain sophisticated answers, ones that incorporate selective arrest strategies and postulate tipping effects and critical masses. I have no trouble believing, given a sophisticated strategy, that the numbers one ends up with can be quite low and still plausibly produce a deterrent effect. I do, however, have a lot of trouble believing that the numbers can plausibly represent anything less than a few million additional arrests per year.

Suppose that to drive down drug use substantially it would be necessary to arrest and meaningfully sanction 20 percent of the people who used drugs during the past year, plus triple the arrests and sanctions of drug dealers. That would mean 5.6 million arrests of users and 951,000 arrests of dealers. To put it another way, arrests of drug users alone—forget the dealers—would be almost twice the number of 1988 arrests for the nation's murders, rapes, robberies, burglaries, aggravated assaults, larcenies, and auto thefts combined.

Now let's think for a moment about what we will do with these people. One may again be open to all sorts of creative penalties and still be unable to imagine how the nation's police and courts can cope with the increased flow of traffic that an effective war on drugs would require. On top of that is the hard truth that an effective deterrent strategy will have to mean incarceration for at least some offenders. If for purposes of illustration we assume that the criminal justice system has to impose some sort of incarceration on 5 percent of the arrested users (which means only 1 percent of all the people who have used drugs during 1988—hardly draconian enforcement) and 75 percent of the arrested dealers, that would come out to a bit less than a million people incarcerated for some period of time. Apart from its sheer size, this number represents more than half again the size of the total 1988 national prison population of 627,000—which was of course already far over the rated capacity of the nation's prisons.

The bottom line is self-evidently ridiculous (though it's not so obvious that the percentages that produced it are ridiculous). Suppose, then, that deterrence can be purchased much more cheaply. First we redefine the number of users to include only those who have used drugs during the past month, not the past year. This cuts the target population by almost half, to 14.5 million. Then we assume that all we have to do to achieve a major deterrent effect on drug use is to arrest 5 percent of these recent users and double the current arrests of dealers. Of the persons arrested, we will incarcerate just 2 percent of the arrested users (meaning just one of every 1,000 recent users overall) and 25 percent of the arrested dealers. This is not "strict law enforcement" by any ordinary definition of "strict," and it is not self-evident that such a policy would raise the risks enough to produce deterrence. The point is that even this optimistic scenario implies that the system somehow has to incarcerate almost 173,000 persons in the first year of the policy, plus arrest and meaningfully punish (short of incarceration) another 1.2 million persons. This bottom line too is ridiculous—and deeply unsettling.

I hold no brief for any of these specific numbers. If you're a hawk and don't like them, change them—but at the end of the line, you have to be able to say, "This will plausibly have a major effect on drug use." I am convinced that punishment can deter drug use, but I cannot figure out how that is to be done in an affordable way, and the hawks have done little to make the case.

Such is the box that I find myself in, perhaps in company with some of my readers. One option, and far from the worst one, is to do nothing more ambitious than we were doing before the War on Drugs began. Drug use in some segments of the population has been dropping for several years. Whatever role the government's drug policy had in this (no one knows), the reductions followed a radical shift in the public perception of drugs. Until the late 1970s, cocaine was still literally fashionable (remember the silver coke spoons worn as jewelry?) among many powerful circles in American society. Since then, drugs have become just as unfashionable in the same circles. Because the opinion leaders don't think it's chic anymore, drug use may well continue to decline no matter what we do.

But to do nothing ignores the toll that drugs and our drug policy are taking on our country. Things aren't necessarily getting better for everyone equally. There are signs that the drug problem is on its way to becoming a manageable problem for the upper classes but not for the lower ones, in the same way that cigarette smoking has plunged in the upper classes and remained virtually unchanged among the lower ones. And though it's all very well to say things will heal themselves sometime in the indefinite future, the problems posed right now are severe, and people whose families are at risk need to be able to do something right now.

Drug-Free Schools

This brings us to the question that should be the starting point in rethinking the drug problem: *What do we really want to accomplish?* By that, I don't mean the usual goals (e.g., "reduce by 50 percent the number of adolescents reporting cocaine use in the past month"). Rather, I am asking you to ask yourself what constitutes "success" regarding the drug problem for you and your family. I also ask you to ignore for the moment that you are affluent or an intellectual or otherwise privileged. What is the selfish solution that would work for you, whether or not it rid the entire nation of drugs?

If you put the goal in this parochial way, some of the answers become relatively simple. Suppose that you are a parent. Your most immediate worry is that your child is going to a school where there is a known drug problem. Step back from the issue, quit brooding about societal ills and complex causes of the national drug problem, and think how absurd it is that the school your child attends has a drug problem. It is not hard for teachers and principals to control schools if they have a free hand to oversee, discipline, suspend, and expel, 1950s-style. Are you willing to give that free hand to your child's school? If yes, then it is easy to run schools so that they have no drug problem, or, more accurately, so that it is no worse than the alcohol problem in the typical 1950s high school.

Consider how drastically the problem of devising good policy changes once the statement of what we are trying to accomplish changes. If I am asked, "Do you have an affordable, practical strategy for reducing adolescent drug use nationwide by 50 percent?"

my honest answer must be no. But if I am asked, "Do you have an affordable practical strategy for sending your child to a school where drugs are not a problem?" my answer is emphatically yes.

The most direct way to achieve this is through a generous, unrestricted voucher program that puts into the hands of parents roughly the current per-pupil costs of public education. Give me the money that my school district currently spends per pupil, do the same for every other parent, and let me choose my own school. If I am really afraid of drugs, I will choose a school with zero tolerance for them—expulsion for the first infraction; frequent, unannounced locker checks; and drug-testing. If I am moderately afraid, I will choose a school with a little more relaxed policy. If I am not afraid at all, I will choose a school where the administration cannot touch my child without due process and a search warrant. Wherever I stand on this spectrum, I know how to send my children to a school that is as drug-free as I wish, and I know how to do so without spending any more money on education or the law enforcement system than we currently spend.

Because most parents probably fall in a mainstream "strict" category, a small minority at either end of the spectrum will have to search for other parents who want drug-permissive environments or maximum-security environments. But this is an immeasurable improvement over the current situation, where millions of families cannot find a school run as they wish. What happens to children who have drug problems? Most of the mainstream schools will refuse to admit them, because to do so would be financially ruinous when the parents of the other children heard about it. That's the virtue of the voucher system. On the other hand, schools that specialize in children with drug problems will mushroom when their parents are carrying around vouchers worth three or four thousand dollars.

Drug-Free Workplaces

I began with the school system because it offers a clear example of the policy revisions I have in mind. But the school example can be generalized. Translated into a policy goal for the War on Drugs, it would read like this: *National drug policy should make it possible for people to send their children to schools that are as drug-free as they wish, live in neighborhoods that are as drug-free as they wish, and work in workplaces that are as drug-free as they wish; and this should apply to poor people as well as rich people, blacks as well as whites, people who live in cities as well as people who live in small towns.*

Forget about eradicating drug use everywhere. If you could live in a neighborhood, work at a job, and send your children to school where drugs weren't a problem—and if everyone else could too if they wanted—wouldn't that pretty much give you what you want in the war against drugs? Let me indicate a few of the ways in which this kind of thinking could apply to the workplace and the neighborhood as well as to schools.

Regarding the workplace, the policy goal is to give employers broad latitude in enforcing drug rules that make sense for that business, and the premise is that the vast majority of businesses have the enlightened self-interest to do just that. Part of my policy prescription is for government to refrain from passing laws about who can and cannot require drug tests. Any employer can make its preferred drug-testing policy a condition of employment. Another part of my policy prescription is specifically to exempt drugs from the tangle of law that currently permits an employee to bring wrongful-discharge suits against an employer. If we're serious about conducting a war on drugs, let employers discharge employees (if they wish—not compulsorily) who test positive for drug use without having to worry about a lawsuit.

It is expensive to get rid of employees who are functioning satisfactorily. This provides a built-in safeguard against arbitrary and abusive behavior by employers—not perfect protection, but a lot of protection. The clear incentive for employers is to establish a policy that lets them act quickly and inexpensively when an employee is exhibiting signs of drug use, with stricter (and more expensive) checks in place only where drug use could endanger people or property. Drug policy would be a matter for collective bargaining agreement in unionized workplaces, and for collaborative development between employees and employers in non-unionized industries. My proposition is that it is just as unnatural for a business to suffer from a debilitating drug problem as it is for a school. It is easy to avoid, in ways that huge majorities of workers and employers can agree upon, if the government and courts will let those workers and employers decide on the conditions of employment without interference.

Drug-Free Neighborhoods

The third sphere within which people should be able to live "as drug-free as they wish"—the neighborhood—would seem to be one place where government enforcement of drug laws is essential unless we want to resort to vigilantism. Nonetheless, bear with me while I postpone calling in the cops and propose a few ways in which we might get to the desired end state without them.

One of the greatly maligned forces for social good in this country is landlords. Whatever their faults, landlords have one undoubted virtue: They want responsible tenants. That is, they want tenants who pay their rent on time and don't trash the property. Given their way, they tend to let good tenants be and to evict bad ones, and this is one of the most efficient forms of socialization known to a free society. Actually, the entire process whereby landlords and tenants find each other is much richer in its social functions than this. Entire neighborhoods represent (or once represented) an intricate process whereby that neighborhood evolved a set of norms and attracted a certain kind of person. Expectations were set up on both sides, and money was often a relatively small part of the discriminating value. In Harlem in the 1940s, for example, the difference between the scruffy, hustling blocks and the exactingly neat and orderly working-class blocks was not a vast difference in income among the tenants, but vast differences in norms and values. In the working-class neighborhoods, unless you presented yourself as being a certain kind of person, you weren't going to get in, even if you could pay the rent. In the scruffy neighborhoods, you could get in, but the landlords charged a premium to compensate for the damage they expected you to cause. Economists have technical descriptions for the equilibria that were reached, but the process was not really so different from the way that human beings everywhere have historically tended to stratify themselves not just according to money, but also according to tastes and values.

In the rush to rid society of the socially disapproved reasons for discriminating among applicants, starting with race, we threw out as well all the ways in which landlords performed a neighborhood-formation function. It became almost impossible for a landlord to say, "I'm not going to rent to you because I don't want you living on my property," which is often what neighborhood-forming decisions have to be based on. Then, ensuring that maintaining cohesive neighborhoods in low-income areas became as difficult as

85

possible, we tore down some of those neighborhoods in the name of urban renewal, threw up public housing in the middle of other such neighborhoods, and in a variety of ways made it impossible for neighborhoods to define and defend themselves.

I realize that getting the government out of the landlord-tenant relationship is an impossibility as of 1990, but a few modest changes might make a big difference. I begin from the observation that the defense of the neighborhood against drugs is a problem especially for black Americans living in urban neighborhoods. The other salient fact is that, in a neighborhood that is already predominantly black, it is difficult for a landlord to discriminate by race. He doesn't get that many opportunities. When a landlord arbitrarily turns down one applicant and chooses another, or when he takes the trouble to evict a tenant (eviction, even without government barriers, is expensive), he is probably doing so for reasons that have nothing to do with race, but a lot to do with trying to get good tenants. Why not free up the housing market in black neighborhoods in the same way that the many "enterprise zone" proposals seek to free up business investment?

I cannot speak to the legal difficulties of drafting the legislation, which might be insurmountable, but the objective is clear enough. In the neighborhoods hardest hit by drugs, make it possible once more for landlords to choose among prospective tenants without having to justify their arbitrariness. If they want to impose a no-drugs rule, they may. If they want to impose a nobody-who-can't-prove-he-has-a-steady-job rule, they may. If they want to impose a no-welfare-mothers rule, they may. If they don't want to rent to you because they don't like your looks, that's up to them. If a tenant violates the terms of the lease, he may be evicted, without the delays that many large cities now superimpose on the terms of the lease. In short, make it possible to make a buck by renting to responsible low-income people. Apply the same freedom to public housing, giving tenant committees wide discretion to screen new applicants and evict existing tenants.

These reforms will permit the creation of neighborhoods of like-minded people in low-income areas. The reason so few white neighborhoods have open-air drug markets is not because police cruisers prowl the streets, but because, for subtler reasons, it would be very foolish for a dealer to set up shop there. For practical purposes, most white neighborhoods already enjoy the same freedoms to form neighborhoods that I propose giving to black neighborhoods. The crazy-quilt of laws and restrictions sometimes gets in the way of middle-class neighborhoods as well, but not often and usually not onerously. The laws and restrictions are really effective in breaking up neighborhoods only when people are poor and where a large proportion of the people rent rather than own. Absent either of those conditions, the attempts of government to interfere with neighborhoods don't work very well, and one or the other is absent in the vast majority of white neighborhoods. Give hardworking, low-income black people the same freedom to segregate themselves into enclaves, using their nonmonetary assets that landlords prize. The aim is not to put all the drug dealers in jail, but to enable people to construct neighborhoods that drug dealers will avoid.

The Power of Communities

This brings us to the question of the underclass. What about the mother who doesn't care what school her children attend? What about the pregnant teenager smoking crack who can't even think far enough ahead to worry about what she's doing to her baby? What about the Uzi-toting young male who has grown up thinking that the way to be a man is to blow away anyone who fails to show him the proper respect? How are school vouchers and a free housing market and employer discretion on drug-testing supposed to do anything for the drug problem in their neighborhoods?

The simplest answer is that maybe it won't do anything at all— but so what? I am not proposing utopia, but a system that enables people to live the kind of life they choose to live. My proposition is that the overwhelming majority of Americans, including the overwhelming majority of low-income black Americans who live in the worst of our inner cities, have sensible preferences about their schools, workplaces, and neighborhoods, and possess the common sense to act on those preferences if we do nothing except make it easier for them to do what they already want to do. I don't know how to turn around the remaining part of the population, but neither do the social engineers. Let us stop fixating on the worst-of-the-worst part of the problem, begin to recognize how badly we have ignored those who are already trying to do everything right, and do the good that we know how to do by helping those who need only a chance. If the result of implementing these policies is to concentrate the bad apples into a few hyper-violent, antisocial neighborhoods, so be it.

In reality, however, I suspect this scenario is too pessimistic. Over a period of time, it seems more plausible that the use of drugs will shrink even among those people who now have the shortest time horizons, the most neglected socialization, and the fewest links with mainstream society. Drug use will drop for essentially the same reason that so many people reading this article have at one time or another taken some kinds of illegal drugs and then stopped with no trouble. It is the reason drug use is dropping in the middle and upper classes. The most profoundly important truth about drugs is not that drugs are evil but that drugs are unsatisfying.

As matters now stand, the choice perceived by many inner-city youths is limited to the life in their streets, drab and dispiriting, compared with the life they see on their television screens, unimaginably glamorous and unattainable. What they badly need are some options closer to home—a neighborhood a few blocks away, not on the other side of town—where the families have fathers as well as mothers, where the streets aren't strewn with garbage, where the playgrounds are safe from gangs and drug dealers. The people in that nearby neighborhood won't necessarily have much more money, for the kinds of qualities I am talking about do not depend on having much money. They depend on the ability of like-minded people to control and shape their small worlds, Burke's little platoons, to the way of life that they prefer. The price of admission to their worlds is not money, but behavior. I submit that, given this visible alternative, large numbers of the people we currently call the underclass eventually will choose to pay that price in return for admission, for the most basic of reasons: the life that people are living in those other neighborhoods really will be richer, more satisfying, more fun, than the life of a drug addict.

All of the effects I have described would probably work better if legalization were added to the package of reforms, but I won't try to make that case here. My more limited point is that the worst of the drug problem will take care of itself if we let the people who want to avoid drugs do so. Enable them to congregate, dominate their neighborhoods, send their children to the same schools. They will set in motion the forces that will bring over a steady stream of converts. To win the war on drugs, it is not necessary that drug abusers become criminals, only that they be made outcasts. In the natural course of events, schools, employees, and communities will do this. Let them.

Appendix: Other Views

A Question of Good Taste
Russell Baker

The idea of legalizing drugs is distasteful for several reasons.

For one, it implies Government approval of addictive, potentially destructive behavior and is, hence, immoral public policy.

True, the Government has legalized alcohol despite its addictive and potentially destructive effects, and people who fret about the immorality of Government alcohol policy are widely thought to be quaint.

True, local governments across the country have legalized gambling, too, despite its well-known addictive and potentially destructive effects.

True, many governments now even run their own legalized versions of what used to be called "the rackets" to lure revenue out of their citizen-suckers.

Complain that this is immoral public policy, and you are likely to be dismissed as a crank or, worse in a society proud of its ruthless pragmatism, as unrealistic about the world we live in.

"You can't stop people from gambling," is the usual explanation, "so why shouldn't the profits go to the state instead of the gangsters?"

True, too, the Government subsidizes the tobacco industry despite its incessantly trumpeted warnings that smoking is addictive and potentially destructive.

The logic of legalized alcohol, legalized gambling and subsidized smoking argues for legalizing drugs. Yet there is very little public support for this logic. The explanation seems to be that there is a stigma attached to drug use and it makes legalizing it too distasteful for Americans to bear.

Smoking, drinking and gambling, whether you call them pleasures or vices, have a long history of being socially acceptable.

Our romantic heroes and heroines have smoked, taken alcohol and gambled for generations. These vices, or pleasures, were certified legalizable by Bette Davis's and Humphrey Bogart's cigarettes, by William Powell's and Myrna Loy's quart-a-day Nick and Nora Charles, by the lovable horse players of "Guys and Dolls," by that ultimate cold war swashbuckler, James Bond.

Drug use has no such glamorous champions unless we go back to Sherlock Holmes. We have no hesitation whether to call it "pleasure" or "vice." All our images of it speak of squalor and death.

"Drugs"—the word summons pictures of dead bodies with needles in their arms, memories of tombstones bearing names like Janis Joplin and Jimi Hendrix. It reminds us of parents numb with grief at their children's graves, of this morning's newspaper pictures of youngsters shot down on the sidewalk.

There is no countervailing association between drugs and wit, charm, fun, good times or romance, as there is in all those old images associated with smoke, booze and gambling. How can anyone propose legalizing something that yields not even a moment of gaiety to balance so much horror?

We are dealing here with a question of esthetics. To the substantial classes who write the laws, drug use is repellent, ugly and nasty.

To substantial people, decent people, ordinary people as they consider themselves, drug use is unredeemed even by such moments of sinful pleasure as they feel in Atlantic City when lighting a cigarette, hoisting a glass of bourbon and putting $100 down on the red.

Americans seem reluctant to admit that their opposition to legalized drugs rests on esthetic objections. They reach for other arguments in an attempt to seem logical.

For instance: the problems created by legalizing one drug (alcohol) are grave enough; why compound them by legalizing others?

This ignores the history of alcohol; to wit, that demand for it has always been so vast in America that the public will create potentially murderous criminal organizations to supply it whenever it is legally unavailable.

Judging from the daily news budget of murder, smuggling, corruption, gang warfare and whole neighborhoods living in terror, demand for drugs now seems so intense that it is not just our own neighborhoods that are imperiled, but the very governments of other nations.

Yet public distaste for drug users is such that few politicians dare discuss whether legalization might be a solution, much less explore what it might require to work effectively.

Instead we get the usual dynamic nonsolutions: more money for weapons to fight a "war on drugs" against the suppliers, more extensions of police power, more muscle, more crackdown.

How all this firepower will reduce the apparently insatiable American demand for drugs is unclear. What is clear is the political strategy: talk bang-bang, get re-elected.

Russell Baker is a columnist for the *New York Times*.
This article is reprinted, with permission, from the *New York Times*, September 6, 1989.

Once Again, a Drug-War Panic

Doug Bandow

Panic is setting in over the mounting toll in the drug war. In an effort to get kids off the streets, the Washington, D.C., city council has voted to join Detroit, Philadelphia and Los Angeles in imposing a curfew on minors. The ordinance (whose enforcement now is blocked by a federal judge's 10-day restraining order) allows the police to stop anyone who looks under 18 and demand his "papers."

If rounding up thousands of kids was not bad enough, many people are demanding that the National Guard, or even the regular Army, be called out to patrol city streets. "Let's declare war," says D.C. council member H. R. Crawford. "We've got to reclaim control of our neighborhoods," writes columnist William Raspberry. Imagine: the nation's capital with armed soldiers on street corners and checkpoints at major intersections.

But then, 44 states are using National Guard units to fight the drug trade in other ways, and the Pentagon is encouraging their efforts, if only to reduce the political pressure on the military to enter the drug war. Nevertheless, drug czar William Bennett reportedly is considering proposals to send U.S. troops into Latin American nations to attack drug laboratories and distribution points.

Even without the help of the National Guard and the military, police across the nation have tried their own versions of "reclaiming control" of the streets. Los Angeles has mounted widespread drives against drug gangs, New York has its Tactical Narcotics Teams and Washington has undertaken Operation Clean Sweep.

However, these campaigns have largely resulted in revolving-door justice. So U.S. Atty. Jay Stephens of the District of Columbia says he may start seeking the death penalty for drug-related murders. But is the killing of a narcotics dealer really worse than the murder of, say, a convenience store clerk?

And how about the punishment for lesser offenders? New York Mayor Ed Koch suggests constructing desert prisons to hold drug dealers, Texas state legislator Al Edwards proposes cutting off a finger for every drug conviction, and Delaware state Sen. Thomas Sharp wants to flog drug felons. Not everyone would hold a trial before inflicting punishment. Two D.C. council members have introduced legislation to pressure landlords to evict accused dealers. New York City already uses a 60-year-old "bawdy house" law for the same purpose, and Peter Vallone, the New York council majority leader, is seeking to extend the principle by seizing the property of people who've merely been indicted for drug offenses.

Of course, potential innocence was never a concern of federal officials when they were promoting their "zero tolerance" campaign last year. You could lose your car if a passenger had a little marijuana. The public outcry, not moral scruples, caused the government to revise its policy.

But these measures pale beside the truly gruesome proposals—to strip-search travelers at the border, gut the 4th Amendment, prosecute the parents of teenage drug users, impose stiff prison sentences for even casual drug use and build a "buried Berlin Wall" along the border with Mexico. Even worse are Customs Commissioner William von Raab's proposal to shoot down the planes of suspected drug smugglers, Sen. Robert Byrd's suggestion that we enlist the KGB (as he put it, "the Soviet Union's worldwide operations and influence") and the bill introduced by Virginia legislators to execute those who sell drugs to minors.

Moreover, the federal government is pressuring private firms, especially government contractors, to adopt drug-testing, one of the most invasive and embarrassing procedures imaginable.

Finally, there is the proposal not only to increase the number of policemen but to increase their incentives to arrest dealers. D.C. Board of Education member R. David Hall has suggested giving cops 10 percent of the booty they seize. Then, he argues, they would become positive role models for youngsters, since they, instead of the dealers, would be profiting from drug sales. In short, join the narcotics squad and get rich.

What sort of society are we becoming? Are we really willing to destroy the nation, or at least the values that make it worth living in, to halt drug use?

Instead of reflexively proposing ever more draconian sanctions, policymakers need to start asking whether the drug war is worth it. Drug abuse ruins lives, but the drug laws and enforcement efforts have become even more destructive. It's time we admitted, as did the nation 56 years ago when it abandoned alcohol prohibition, that the cost of trying to protect people from themselves is simply too high.

Doug Bandow is a senior fellow at the Cato Institute and a nationally syndicated columnist.
This article is reprinted, with permission, from the *Chicago Tribune*, March 22, 1989.

We Need a Legalization "Fix"

Randy E. Barnett and Tom G. Palmer

Each year Americans spend more and more money to maintain a self-destructive habit. As the horrible effects of this habit become more and more apparent, Americans engage in ever more tortuous acts of denial, confident that just another "fix" will make the nightmares go away.

The addiction is not to drugs. It is to drug laws.

The simple fact is that America's second experiment with prohibition is ending—like the first—in complete failure at a terrible cost. Drug prohibition has introduced millions of Americans to lives of crime and violence. Prohibition has multiplied prices on the black market a thousand-fold or more, leading drug addicts to commit crimes against the rest of us—and each other—to get the money to support their habits. Prohibition has let punks get rich controlling the drug markets, corrupting law enforcement agencies in the United States and governments overseas in the process.

Are drug laws supposed to help the addicts? As harmful as using drugs may be to someone, being imprisoned makes matters much worse. And drug peddlers can hardly be prevented from selling adulterated and poisoned drugs that kill their customers—sometimes on purpose—leaving addicts at the mercy of unaccountable and unscrupulous suppliers.

Are drug laws supposed to protect the nondrug-using majority from the addicts? As disheartening as it may be to know that another person is harming himself with drugs (or alcohol or tobacco), it is even worse to be robbed or burgled by an addict who cannot otherwise afford artificially expensive drugs.

Are drug laws supposed to keep drugs away from young people? Black-market prices and profit margins created by drug laws have encouraged sellers to seek customers among the most impressionable and gullible—our children. Indeed, children are the most effective sellers to other children. Those seeking the illegal "thrill" of marijuana are driven into contact with some of the most violent criminals our society has ever produced. There is no evidence that marijuana necessarily leads to "harder stuff," but there is evidence that becoming involved with drug dealers does.

Drug laws also are responsible for the ever-increasing potency and dangerousness of illegal drugs. Making comparatively benign, grown drugs such as opiates artificially scarce creates powerful (black) market incentives for clandestine chemists to develop alternative "synthetic" drugs—PCP, for example—that can be made more cheaply and with less risk of detection by law enforcement. But these drugs can be far more dangerous than the substances they replace, both to the user and to others.

Drug laws have helped to turn cities into combat zones, as addicts rob the public for money, dealers rob customers, customers rob dealers and rival gangs shoot it out over control of turf. About half the murder cases one of us (Barnett) prosecuted as assistant state's attorney for Cook County, Ill., were "drug related"—the victim was killed because he was thought to have either drugs or money from the sale of drugs.

Crimes also are committed against persons who seek out criminals from whom to purchase illegal drugs. In one case, three young men who sought to buy marijuana from street gang members were brutally stabbed to death because, in seeking to gain the gang members' trust, they unknowingly aligned themselves with a rival gang. Strictly speaking, drug laws "worked" in this case. The gang had no marijuana for sale, and the kids didn't get high.

This mess is not just a horrible accident to be solved by more money, better personnel and tougher penalties. It is an unavoidable consequence of prohibiting conduct that is "victimless"—not in the sense that no one is harmed but in the narrower sense that there is no victim to report a crime or infraction, or to testify at the trial. This lack of a *complaining* victim is important for understanding the effects of drug laws.

Without a complaining victim, enforcement depends on the most intrusive of police techniques—searches, drug tests, criminal informants. Moreover, with no complainant, prosecution depends on police initiative and testimony, giving rise to enormous opportunities for corruption by "looking the other way." And drug busts are quite effective in enforcing the extortion of bribes.

The incentives created by making drug use illegal are perverse when compared to a crime—such as robbery—with a complaining victim. Robbery laws reduce the profit that sellers of illegally obtained goods receive by forcing robbers who take anything but cash to sell their booty at a tremendous discount. Drug laws, however, have the opposite effect. They create an artificial scarcity of a *desired* product. Willing buyers pay sellers grossly higher prices than they would without such laws.

While the threat of punishment makes being a drug supplier more costly, this cost is more than offset by reducing the risk of capture (payoffs to the police), by increasing the return (higher prices) and by attracting sellers who are less "risk averse"—people who live only for today with nothing to lose if caught. That is why drug suppliers are typically evil, violent and dangerous people while the corner liquor store clerk is not.

Yet there is another futile effort being made to satisfy our insatiable and dangerous addiction to drug prohibition. Prominent politicians are urging that the U.S. Army be deployed to "wipe out" drugs (inevitably resulting in the corruption of the Army), that the Air Force shoot down planes "suspected" of carrying illegal drugs (inevitably resulting in the death of innocents), that everyone's urine be subjected to random compulsory tests (resulting in careers and lives ruined by inevitable false-positive results) and that the death penalty be imposed for sale of drugs (inevitably resulting in heightened violence against the police and their informants).

It is time to question whether the next stage in our costly "war on drugs" is just another "fix." It is time to go cold turkey. It is time to legalize illegal drugs.

Randy E. Barnett is a professor at the Illinois Institute of Technology, Chicago-Kent College of Law, and a former Cook County prosecutor. Tom G. Palmer is a fellow at the Institute for Humane Studies at George Mason University.
This article is reprinted, with permission, from the *Detroit News*, May 20, 1988.

Let's Quit the Drug War

David Boaz

An antiwar song that helped get the Smothers Brothers thrown off network television in the 60's went this way: "We're waist deep in the Big Muddy, and the big fool says to push on." Today we're waist-deep in another unwinnable war, and many political leaders want to push on. This time it's a war on drugs. About 23 million Americans use illicit drugs every month, despite annual Federal outlays of $3.9 billion. Even the arrests of 824,000 Americans a year don't seem to be having much effect.

As in the case of Vietnam—and Prohibition, another unwinnable war—many politicians can't stand losing a war. Instead of acknowledging failure, they want to escalate.

Mayor Edward I. Koch of New York suggests that we strip search every person entering the United States from Mexico or Southeast Asia. The White House drug adviser, Donald I. MacDonald, calls for arresting even small-time users—lawyers with a quarter-gram of cocaine, high school kids with a couple of joints—and bringing them before a judge.

Where will we put those two-bit "criminals"? The Justice Department recommends doubling our prison capacity, even though President Reagan's former drug adviser Carlton E. Turner already brags about the role of drug laws in bringing about a 60 percent increase in our prison population in the last six years. Bob Dole calls for the death penalty for drug sellers.

Like their counterparts in Los Angeles and Chicago, the Washington, D.C., police are to be issued semiautomatic pistols so they can engage in ever bloodier shootouts with drug dealers. Members of the District of Columbia Council call for the National Guard to occupy the city. We've already pressed other governments to destroy drug crops and to help us interdict the flow of drugs into the United States. Because those measures have largely failed, the Customs Service asks authorization to "use appropriate force" to compel planes *suspected* of carrying drugs to land, including the authority to shoot them down.

It's time to ask ourselves: What kind of society would condone strip searches, large-scale arrests, military occupation of its capital city and the shooting of possibly innocent people in order to stop some of its citizens from using substances that others don't like?

Prohibition of alcohol in the 1920's failed because it proved impossible to stop people from drinking. Our 70-year effort at prohibition of marijuana, cocaine and heroin has also failed. Tens of millions of Americans, including senators, Presidential candidates, a Supreme Court nominee and conservative journalists, have broken the laws against such drugs. Preserving laws that are so widely flouted undermines respect for all laws.

The most dangerous drugs in the United States are alcohol, which is responsible for about 100,000 deaths a year, and tobacco, which is responsible for about 350,000. Heroin, cocaine and marijuana account for a total of 3,600 deaths a year—even though one in five people aged 20 to 40 uses drugs regularly.

Our efforts to crack down on illegal drug use have created new problems. A Justice Department survey reports that 70 percent of those arrested for serious crimes are drug users, which may mean that "drugs cause crime." A more sophisticated analysis suggests that the high cost of drugs, a result of their prohibition, forces drug users to turn to crime to support an unnecessarily expensive habit.

Drug prohibition, by giving young people the thrill of breaking the law and giving pushers a strong incentive to find new customers, may actually increase the number of drug users. Moreover, our policy of pressuring friendly governments to wipe out drug cultivation has undermined many of those regimes and provoked resentment against us among their citizens and government officials.

We can either escalate the war on drugs, which would have dire implications for civil liberties and the right to privacy, or find a way to gracefully withdraw. Withdrawal should not be viewed as an endorsement of drug use; it would simply be an acknowledgment that the cost of this war—billions of dollars, runaway crime rates and restrictions on our personal freedom—is too high.

David Boaz is executive vice president of the Cato Institute.

This article is reprinted, with permission, from the *New York Times*, March 17, 1988.

Legalize Dope

William F. Buckley, Jr.

We are with reason angry at the Mexican officials who ho-hummed their way through an investigation of the torture and killing of a U.S. drug agent. It is true that a few years ago the government of Mexico cooperated in a program designed to spray the marijuana crop, but it proved temporary. Somewhat like wage and price controls. If for a season the marijuana crop from Mexico declines, then marijuana from elsewhere—Hawaii, for instance—will increase. If there is less marijuana being smoked today than 10 years ago, it is a reflection not of law enforcement but of creeping social perception. It has gradually transpired that the stuff is more harmful than originally thought, and a culture that spends billions of dollars on health foods and barbells is taking a longer, critical look at marijuana.

We read about cocaine. In a vivid image, someone recently said that the big radars along the 2,000-mile border between Mexico and the United States begin, night after night, to track what looks like a swarm of locusts headed our way. Private planes, carrying coke to the American market.

So we bag a large number of them today, and they show up on the television news. That plane over there was carrying $10 million (or was it $100 million?) worth of coke, hurray for the Drug Enforcement Agency. But then the sober evaluation comes through. Last year—a splendid year for drug apprehension—resulted in interdicting, oh, maybe 10 percent, 20 percent of the stuff coming in.

And of course the measure of success in the drug business, like that in the business of robbing banks, is, what are your chances of getting through? Answer: terrific. The odds will always be high, when you consider that the amount of coke you can stuff into a single pocket of a man's jacket can fetch $200,000, and that the cost of the stuff where picked up can be as low as $1,000. A profit of 2,000 percent (modest in the business) is a powerful engine to try to stop in a free society.

So what are we going to do about it? My resourceful brother William Safire has a hot bundle of ideas aimed at catching the people who launder the profits from drugs. These ideas include changing the color of our currency, so that the boys with big sackfuls of green under their mattresses will be forced to bring them out, revealing their scarlet letters. Maybe we should breed 50 million drug-trained dogs to sniff at everyone getting off a boat or an airplane; what a great idea!

No, we are face to face with the rawest datum of them all, which is that the problem would not exist, except that in the United States there is a market for the stuff, and that the stuff is priced very high. If we cannot effectively prevent its insinuating its way into the country, what is it that we can prevent? The answer, of course, is its price. The one thing that could be done, overnight, is to legalize the stuff. Exit crime, and the profits from vice.

It is hardly a novel suggestion to legalize dope. Shrewd observers of the scene have recommended it for years. I am on record as having opposed it in the matter of heroin. The accumulated evidence draws me away from my own opposition, on the purely empirical grounds that what we have now is a drug problem plus a crime problem plus a problem of a huge export of capital to the dope-producing countries.

Congress should study the dramatic alternative, which is legalization followed by a dramatic educational effort in which the services of all civic-minded, and some less than civic-minded, resources are mobilized.

Ours is a free society in which oodles of people kill themselves with tobacco and booze. Some will do so with coke and heroin. But we should count in the lives saved by having the deadly stuff available at the same price as rat poison.

William F. Buckley, Jr., is editor-in-chief of *National Review* and a nationally syndicated columnist.

This article is reprinted, with permission, from the *Washington Post*, April 1, 1985.

We're Losing the Drug War Because Prohibition Never Works

Hodding Carter III

There is clearly no point in beating a dead horse, whether you are a politician or a columnist, but sometimes you have to do it just the same, if only for the record. So, for the record, here's another attempt to argue that a majority of the American people and their elected representatives can be and are wrong about the way they have chosen to wage the "war against drugs." Prohibition can't work, won't work and has never worked, but it can and does have monumentally costly effects on the criminal justice system and on the integrity of government at every level.

Experience should be the best teacher, and my experience with prohibition is a little more recent than that of most Americans for whom the "noble experiment" ended with repeal in 1933. In my home state of Mississippi, it lasted for an additional 33 years, and for all those years it was a truism that the drinkers had their liquor, the preachers had their prohibition and the sheriffs made the money. Al Capone would have been proud of the latitude that bootleggers were able to buy with their payoffs of constables, deputies, police chiefs and sheriffs across the state.

But as a first-rate series in the *New York Times* made clear early last year, Mississippi's prohibition-era corruption (and Chicago's before that) was penny ante stuff compared with what is happening in the U.S. today. From Brooklyn police precincts to Miami's police stations to rural Georgia courthouses, big drug money is purchasing major breakdowns in law enforcement. Sheriffs, other policemen and now judges are being bought up by the gross. But that money, with the net profits for the drug traffickers estimated at anywhere from $40 billion to $100 billion a year, is also buying up banks, legitimate businesses and to the south of us, entire governments. The latter becomes an increasingly likely outcome in a number of cities and states in this country as well. Cicero, Ill., during Prohibition is an instructive case in point.

The money to be made from an illegal product that has about 23 million current users in this country also explains why its sale is so attractive on the mean streets of America's big cities. A street salesman can gross about $2,500 a day in Washington, which puts him in the pay category of a local television anchor, and this in a neighborhood of dead-end job chances.

Since the courts and jails are already swamped beyond capacity by the arrests that are routinely made (44,000 drug dealers and users over a two-year period in Washington alone, for instance) and since those arrests barely skim the top of the pond, arguing that stricter enforcement is the answer begs a larger question: Who is going to pay the billions of dollars required to build the prisons, hire the judges, train the policemen and employ the prosecutors needed for the load already on hand, let alone the huge one yet to come if we ever get serious about arresting dealers and users?

Much is made of the costs of drug addiction, and it should be, but the current breakdown in the criminal justice system is not one of them. That breakdown is the result of prohibition, not addiction. Drug addiction, after all, does not come close to the far vaster problems of alcohol and tobacco addiction (as former Surgeon General Koop correctly noted, tobacco is at least as addictive as heroin).

103

Hard drugs are estimated to kill 4,000 people a year directly and several tens of thousands a year indirectly. Alcohol kills at least 100,000 a year, addicts millions more and costs the marketplace billions of dollars. Tobacco kills over 300,000 a year, addicts tens of millions and fouls the atmosphere as well. But neither alcohol nor tobacco threatens to subvert our system of law and order, because they are treated as personal and societal problems rather than as criminal ones.

Indeed, every argument that is made for prohibiting the use of currently illegal drugs can be made even more convincingly about tobacco and alcohol. The effects on the unborn? Staggeringly direct. The effects on adolescents? Alcoholism is the addiction of choice for young Americans on a ratio of about 100 to one. Lethal effect? Tobacco's murderous results are not a matter of debate anywhere outside the Tobacco Institute.

Which leaves the lingering and legitimate fear that legalization might produce a surge in use. It probably would, although not nearly as dramatic a one as opponents usually estimate. The fact is that personal use of marijuana, whatever the local laws may say, has been virtually decriminalized for some time now, but there has been a stabilization or slight decline in use, rather than an increase, for several years. Heroin addiction has held steady at about 500,000 people for some time, though the street price of heroin is far lower now than it used to be. Use of cocaine in its old form also seems to have stopped climbing and begun to drop off among young and old alike, though there is an abundantly available supply.

That leaves crack cocaine, stalker of the inner city and terror of the suburbs. Instant and addictive in effect, easy to use and relatively cheap to buy, it is a personality-destroying substance that is a clear menace to its users. But it is hard to imagine it being any more accessible under legalization than it is in most cities today under prohibition, while the financial incentives for promoting its use would virtually disappear with legalization.

Proponents of legalization should not try to fuzz the issue, nonetheless. Addiction levels might increase, at least temporarily, if legal sanctions were removed. That happened after the repeal of Prohibition, or so at least some studies have suggested. But while that would be a personal disaster for the addicts and their families, and would involve larger costs to society as a whole, those costs

104

would be minuscule compared with the costs of continued prohibition.

The young Capones of today own the inner cities and the wholesalers behind these young retailers are rapidly buying up the larger system which is supposed to control them. Prohibition gave us the Mafia and organized crime on a scale that has been with us ever since. The new prohibition is writing a new chapter on that old text. Hell-bent on learning nothing from history, we are witnessing its repetition, predictably enough, as tragedy.

Hodding Carter III is a political commentator who heads a television production firm.

This article is reprinted, with permission, from the *Wall Street Journal*, July 13, 1989.

Nancy Reagan and the Real Villains in the Drug War
Stephen Chapman

"The casual user may think when he takes a line of cocaine or smokes a joint in the privacy of his nice condo, listening to his expensive stereo, that he's somehow not bothering anyone. But there is a trail of death and destruction that leads directly to his door. I'm saying that if you're a casual drug user, you are an accomplice to murder."

That was Nancy Reagan's latest broadside against drug use. It was certainly timely. A few days earlier, a New York City policeman, assigned to guard a man who had been threatened by drug dealers, was shot to death in his patrol car. The nation's capital is being terrorized by a wave of drug-related killings. Just a few weeks ago, the attorney general of Colombia was murdered, apparently in revenge for his campaign against the nation's cocaine cartel.

But neither the First Lady nor anyone else in the government appears ready for a remedy that might actually put a stop to incidents like these. Despite the apparent urgency of the problem and the fierce rhetoric, the only proposal is more of the same.

A 20-year war on drugs, which has been escalated by this administration, has done nothing to make us safer. Only one policy offers any hope of improvement: to stop treating people who use or sell illicit drugs as criminals.

Americans forget that there is a precedent for this crisis. During the 1920s, cities like Chicago served as battlefields for a grim war between criminals and police. In one three-year stretch, the violence here claimed the lives of more than 400 criminals and police officers. Between 1920 and 1933, New York City and more than 1,000 gangland murders.

The cause of all this was a war on another drug—alcohol. The roots of the violence lay not in the inherent qualities of alcohol, but in its prohibition. Likewise, what spurs the bloodshed in the drug trade is not the drugs, but the attempt to suppress them. What ended the Prohibition-era violence was the legalization of alcohol. Today, distillers and liquor store owners don't fight for market share with machine guns.

In some places, especially Washington, D.C., drug-related crime is an epidemic. In 1985, the capital had 25 drug-related murders. In 1987, there were 130. In the first two months of 1988, at least 42 people have died in such episodes, double the rate last year. Other crimes in the capital show the same trend. The number of indictments on drug-related felonies has risen sevenfold since 1982.

These developments happened even as the administration was mounting its anti-drug offensive, which has accomplished little in slowing the flow. The *Washington Post* reports that cocaine use "is up, inventories are high, prices are down and the cocaine sold on the street has never been higher." When New York Democrat Charles Rangel, chairman of the House Select Committee on Narcotics Abuse and Control, was asked about advances in halting drug traffic, he replied, "We haven't made any."

While drug use persists, the illegal commerce in drugs has gotten more violent. Execution-style slayings now dominate the news in Washington, where the crime wave springs from an attempt by Jamaican drug gangs to seize a share of the business, something resisted by established dealers.

A police spokesman in suburban Prince George's County, Maryland, explained it: "When you're an outsider, you have to cut yourself a piece of the territory that's already owned by someone else. How do you do it? You start shooting."

The pathology exactly matches that of Prohibition. By making drugs illegal, the government raises their price. That makes them more profitable. The more profitable they are, the more attractive to those suppliers who are willing to use illegal and even violent methods to sell them.

Raising the price also incites crime of another sort. Addicts who need hundreds of dollars a day to finance their addictions have few options but to steal. So it's not surprising to discover, as a recent Justice Department study did, that some 70 percent of the people arrested for serious crimes are drug users. The lesson is not that drug use itself causes larceny and violence, but that the illegality of these drugs pushes users into other, more serious types of crime.

Legalizing the illicit drugs that have been the object of so much hysteria may sound like a drastic step. Nothing else, though, holds any prospect of restoring a measure of security to our cities.

Nancy Reagan and the other crusaders against drugs may continue to preach that still tougher measures are needed. But no one should imagine they will succeed at anything but perpetuating the bloody status quo. And no one should have any doubt who are the real accomplices to murder.

Stephen Chapman is a nationally syndicated columnist.
This article is reprinted, with permission, from the *Chicago Tribune*, March 6, 1988.

Legalizing Drugs—Step No. 1

Kildare Clarke

In December 1988, I pronounced the death by gunshot of an 18-year-old Hispanic male as his younger brother sobbed and his mother looked on in great pain. This is nothing out of the ordinary for a physician at Kings County Hospital, located in one of New York City's drug combat zones, the Flatbush section of Brooklyn.

Six months later, the same mother looked on as I pronounced the death by gunshot wound of the son who had earlier sobbed at his older brother's death. He was 17, and had $7,000 in his pocket. No one had to ask where he got the money.

Increasingly, the emergency room at Kings County Hospital has the feel of a MASH unit. The battered bodies and broken dreams that pass through every day and night are constant reminders that we have lost the conventional war against drugs.

The users, of course, are not the only ones who end up in the emergency room. Drug-related violence has escalated to the point where innocent victims are shot every week, and not-so-innocent drug dealers and aspiring dealers are killed at a rate of about three a day.

Most of these deaths come early to young men who could have been leaders in the city. But instead of pursuing educational avenues, which take time to produce rewards, they turn to the more profitable and alluring business of dealing drugs.

And that's the real drug problem: profits, and the power and respect that come with them. As the mayoral campaign has progressed, I have searched for some recognition by the candidates of this fundamental truth. Instead, I hear promises to clean up the streets using the same failed approaches: more Federal dollars, more police officers, more judges and more prison cells.

To those of us near the front lines, such proposals ring hollow. Obviously, the lure of making fast nontaxable money through the illegal drug trade far outweighs the risk not only of prison but of death.

I realize that no one gets elected to public office by taking the wrong side of controversial issues. But I also know that myopia rarely lends itself to great leadership. If the candidates were as serious about ending the drug war as they profess to be, then they would at least discuss the option of legalizing drugs, which is the first step toward a sensible drug policy.

We have to see the drug problem clearly, without emotion. Drugs—or, more specifically, drug profits—are the linchpin of our most vexing urban problems: crime, homelessness and the breakdown of the family.

Look at the benefits of legalization. By removing black-market profits, it would substantially reduce the violence that goes with the illegal trade and the street crime that supports drug habits. It would stop the killing of police officers and innocent bystanders caught in the crossfire. It would allow better controls, reducing the chance of death by overdose or transmission of AIDS by dirty needles.

The beneficial effects on communities and families would be just as pronounced. We could re-establish good role models and preserve our future leaders. Parents, who too often now take orders from their drug-wealthy children, would have greater authority to discipline their kids and convince them to remain in school.

We need to ask the candidates: How long should the citizens of New York City and the country as a whole continue to live under the drug cartels' dictatorial rule?

How many more Maria Hernandezes or Officer Byrneses must we mourn before the truth about our failed policy is recognized?

Must we wait until millions of lives are lost before we arrive at the foregone conclusion that the legalization of drugs is the only solution to the problem?

Would legalization cause an increase in drug use? Yes, initially, it probably would. However, education and treatment, where necessary, would be part of the package.

Compare drugs and alcohol. We have many problem drinkers, and alcohol abuse is of concern to us all. But since the end of Prohibition, we have not had to contend with organized killing for control of the trade. Today, we are educating the public about the long-term effects of alcohol, providing treatment for those in need and, overall, dealing with alcohol in a far more rational fashion than we are coping with drugs.

By far the most dramatic result of legalization would be the drop in drug-related crime and violence. The money we now spend on controlling and criminalizing drugs could be spent on any number of things—from education to low-income housing to law enforcement—to further enhance the safety of our streets.

No single step could do more to improve the quality of life in New York City than to legalize drugs. The real question is, why don't the candidates at least talk about it?

Kildare Clarke is associate medical director of the emergency department of Kings County Hospital in Brooklyn.

This article is reprinted, with permission, from the *New York Times*, August 26, 1989.

Why Not Try Decriminalization?

Richard Cohen

The *Economist*, a well-respected British news magazine, is regarded as right of center. The *National Review* is, of course, the magazine founded by William F. Buckley Jr., and to say it's right of center is like saying it's cold in Siberia. What, besides politics, do these publications have in common? Both have proposed the decriminalization of drugs.

What? I hear you say. But you thought this was only Cohen's crackpot idea. Pray, no. Support has come from the most unlikely quarters, some of it giving me second thoughts. My God, I say, if Buckley has been wrong about so much, why should this issue be any different?

And in truth I can't be sure it is. The decriminalization of drugs would be a leap into the unknown. No one knows what would happen. We do know, however, what the situation is now, and we have it on the testimony of some of the leading drug busters in the land (Secretary of Education William Bennett, former President Nixon) that we are losing the war. To hear them tell it, the situation is out of control.

Maybe. But one thing that's out of control is the rhetoric politicians use about drugs. Everyone wants to use the military to seal our borders, although no one knows quite how this would be done—or at what cost. Nixon, who launched the so-called War on Drugs, is one of those calling for the Army. He forgets that in Vietnam 500,000 troops could not seal South Vietnam from North Vietnam. (Maybe he wants to bomb Colombia, as he did Cambodia?)

Nixon, in fact, personifies the approach the country has taken to drugs. Appearing on "Meet the Press" Sunday, he used the direst language to describe the problem: "The purpose of our armed forces is to deal with an enemy of the United States. And, believe me, those that engage in selling drugs . . . are killing people just as much as an enemy does."

Oh, yeah, how many people? The figure supplied by Ethan Nadelmann in *Foreign Policy* magazine is 3,562 for all drugs in 1985. Nadelmann, a Princeton University professor, compares illicit drugs with two licit ones: alcohol and tobacco. Alcohol, he says, was the "direct cause" of 80,000 to 100,000 deaths and "a contributing cause" of an additional 100,000. As for tobacco, Nadelmann cites 1984 figures: 320,000 deaths.

Of course, fatalities are not the only cost to society of drugs. Crime is another. But Nadelmann's comparison is apt. The United States has come to terms with alcohol. After Prohibition failed, the drug was decriminalized. We distinguish between alcohol consumption and abuse, set standards for its manufacture (when you buy Scotch, you get Scotch) and place restrictions on it, such as prohibiting its sale to minors. The system has not worked perfectly (there are about 18 million alcohol abusers or alcoholics) and maybe not even well, but realism has prevailed: we live with alcohol.

Decriminalization of drugs might bring about the same result. We would still have addicts. We would still have a drug problem. Kids would manage to get their hands on drugs—just as they do booze. But we would learn to distinguish between use and abuse and between different drugs. (Marijuana, for instance, kills no one, but it's sometimes sold by dealers who have an incentive to encourage heroin use.) The government could set standards so that overdoses would be rare and—most important—reduce the price of the stuff so that it would no longer be such a profitable enterprise for criminals. Say what you will about the decriminalization of alcohol, it has rid the nation of bootleggers.

There is really no such thing as a victimless crime. But crimes in which the victim is complicitous are almost impossible to eradicate. A robbery victim will call the police; a drug buyer will not. Crackdowns invariably result in the action's being moved elsewhere—up the street in the case of street sales, from Florida to Texas when it comes to drug smuggling. Except in encouraging criminal activity, the current drug policy has been a bust.

Illicit drugs are a public health problem. So is alcohol. But unlike alcohol, drugs are treated primarily as a criminal problem. The remedy proposed by most politicians amounts to more of the same: more police, more military, more and stiffer jail sentences. In Medellin, Colombia, the drug czars must be laughing themselves sick. They can get high just on the pronouncements of American politicians.

Failure is a bitter pill, but once it is taken, at least we can move on. When I called the *National Review* to check my memory ("Did you really endorse the decriminalization of drugs?"), I was told "endorse" was not the right word. "Propose" was—as in "it's worth thinking about." My sentiments exactly.

Richard Cohen is a columnist for the *Washington Post*.
This article is reprinted, with permission, from the *Washington Post*, April 12, 1988.

Mission Impossible
The Economist

With two centuries of prosperous and stable democracy behind it, the government of the United States of America has failed to master its national curse of drugs and drug-financed crime. Colombia, a poor apprentice democracy with a horrendous history of violence, has better excuses for its more abject failure. Yet both, in their different ways, are failing for the same reason: what they are trying to do is incapable of success. Repression, however vigorous, cannot win the war against drugs. It is time to try a better way.

Nobody can accuse the Colombian government of faintheartedness. For most of last month drug dealers were murdering yet more of their arch-enemies, the country's honest judges, policemen and political hopefuls. President Virgilio Barco deployed his powers under the 30-year-old state of emergency to order the arbitrary arrest of 11,000 people, the sequestration of millions of dollars' worth of property, and the extradition without due process of suspects to face trial in the United States. But the big birds, alerted by their corrupted informers in the government services, had flown.

Most of those captured, and most of the seized property, will be released for lack of proof of their guilty associations. Of the 89 people whose extradition the United States most pressingly seeks, only one mere book-keeper awaits the flight northwards. The big traders ordered their henchmen to bomb some banks and government buildings, then slipped across the borders to well prepared retreats and to the Panamanian bank-branches where their money sits secure. Cocaine traders are the world's richest businessmen.

Out of their tax-free profits they outspend, outnumber and outgun the law-enforcement powers of poor states, and dent the civil peace and dignity of the world's richest nation too.

President Bush has responded promptly to Mr Barco's bravery, digging into the Pentagon's reserves to send helicopters, small-arms and other weapons. This support was unusually swift and well calculated (and delivered without pious advice); it was followed by promises of more generous economic aid. Attacking foreign drug-suppliers fits well with the new domestic policy that the president and his "drug tsar," Mr William Bennett, are soon to announce. Americans want a response to the inter-gang shoot-outs in their cities and the wholesale poisoning of young men, women and unborn children. The new offensive promises to be more comprehensive and much more expensive than the rag-tag skirmishes that have preceded it. But it stands little more chance of success than Mr Barco's more desperate endeavour. To understand why, Americans need only look back at their own country's not-too-distant history.

From 1920 until 1933, American citizens were forbidden to buy or sell their favourite dangerous drug, alcohol. The beer-trucks and the whiskey-schooners kept on coming, creating what were then the most profitable criminal organisations in the world. Now mankind has developed the appetite for yet more powerful drugs, and subjected them to a wider and equally fruitless ban.

Drugs are bad for people. They should not want them—legal alcohol and tobacco, illegal heroin, cocaine, marijuana, or cheap and risky "designer" substitutes dreamt up by artful chemists. Yet demand creates supply, despite the panoply of international conventions and national laws whose main effect is to create still vaster profits for the traders. The drug exporters of Latin America—and of Lebanon, Pakistan, the Burma-Thailand golden triangle and the rest—buy up or terrorise governments, and defy even so-far-uncorrupted regimes, just as North America's mafias, yard-crowds and cartels defy the will of Washington.

As long as people spend money for a thrill, prohibition cannot work. It turns an issue of personal choice and health into a crisis of criminality. Governments protect drinkers by quality controls, taxes and licensing that divert demand away from the most destructive forms of booze. For cigarette smokers, governments insist on health

113

warnings. To protect people against damage from bad food or therapeutic drugs, they test and measure the products' effects. Illegal drugs they merely outlaw and, while failing to enforce the outlawry, forgo the power to regulate the trade.

Prohibition, and its inevitable failure, make a bad business more criminal, more profitable and more dangerous to its customers than it need be. Lifting the ban, and replacing it with detailed regulation, might certainly expose more people to risky experiments with drugs. That danger is real—even if experience shows that relatively few people are foolish enough to go beyond experiments.

But prohibition's failure is more dangerous yet, both for individual drug-takers and for societies corrupted, subverted and terrorised by the drug gangs. The trade is banned by national laws and international conventions. Repeal them, replace them by control, taxation and discouragement. Until that is done, the slaughter in the United States, and the destruction of Colombia, will continue. Europe's turn is next.

This article is reprinted, with permission, from the *Economist*, September 2, 1989.

An Open Letter to Bill Bennett

Milton Friedman

Dear Bill:

In Oliver Cromwell's eloquent words, "I beseech you, in the bowels of Christ, think it possible you may be mistaken" about the course you and President Bush urge us to adopt to fight drugs. The path you propose of more police, more jails, use of the military in foreign countries, harsh penalties for drug users, and a whole panoply of repressive measures can only make a bad situation worse. The drug war cannot be won by those tactics without undermining the human liberty and individual freedom that you and I cherish.

You are not mistaken in believing that drugs are a scourge that is devastating our society. You are not mistaken in believing that drugs are tearing asunder our social fabric, ruining the lives of many young people, and imposing heavy costs on some of the most disadvantaged among us. You are not mistaken in believing that the majority of the public share your concerns. In short, you are not mistaken in the end you seek to achieve.

Your mistake is failing to recognize that the very measures you favor are a major source of the evils you deplore. Of course the problem is demand, but it is not only demand, it is demand that must operate through repressed and illegal channels. Illegality creates obscene profits that finance the murderous tactics of the drug lords; illegality leads to the corruption of law enforcement officials; illegality monopolizes the efforts of honest law forces so that they are starved for resources to fight the simpler crimes of robbery, theft and assault.

Drugs are a tragedy for addicts. But criminalizing their use converts that tragedy into a disaster for society, for users and non-users alike. Our experience with the prohibition of drugs is a replay of our experience with the prohibition of alcoholic beverages.

I wrote a column in 1972 on "Prohibition and Drugs." The major problem then was heroin from Marseilles; today, it is cocaine from Latin America. Today, also, the problem is far more serious than it was 17 years ago: more addicts, more innocent victims; more drug pushers, more law enforcement officials; more money spent to enforce prohibition, more money spent to circumvent prohibition.

Had drugs been decriminalized 17 years ago, "crack" would never have been invented (it was invented because the high cost of illegal drugs made it profitable to provide a cheaper version) and there would today be far fewer addicts. The lives of thousands, perhaps hundreds of thousands of innocent victims would have been saved, and not only in the U.S. The ghettos of our major cities would not be drug-and-crime-infested no-man's lands. Fewer people would be in jails, and fewer jails would have been built.

Colombia, Bolivia and Peru would not be suffering from narco-terror, and we would not be distorting our foreign policy because of narco-terror. Hell would not, in the words with which Billy Sunday welcomed Prohibition, "be forever for rent," but it would be a lot emptier.

Decriminalizing drugs is even more urgent now than in 1972, but we must recognize that the harm done in the interim cannot be wiped out, certainly not immediately. Postponing decriminalization will only make matters worse, and make the problem appear even more intractable.

Alcohol and tobacco cause many more deaths in users than do drugs. Decriminalization would not prevent us from treating drugs as we now treat alcohol and tobacco: prohibiting sales of drugs to minors, outlawing the advertising of drugs and similar measures. Such measures could be enforced, while outright prohibition cannot be. Moreover, if even a small fraction of the money we now spend on trying to enforce drug prohibition were devoted to treatment and rehabilitation, in an atmosphere of compassion not punishment, the reduction in drug usage and in the harm done to the users could be dramatic.

This plea comes from the bottom of my heart. Every friend of freedom, and I know you are one, must be as revolted as I am by the prospect of turning the United States into an armed camp, by the vision of jails filled with casual drug users and of an army of enforcers empowered to invade the liberty of citizens on slight evidence. A country in which shooting down unidentified planes "on suspicion" can be seriously considered as a drug-war tactic is not the kind of United States that either you or I want to hand on to future generations.

Milton Friedman is a senior research fellow at the Hoover Institution and a Nobel laureate in economics.

This article is reprinted, with permission, from the *Wall Street Journal*, September 7, 1989.

Treat It like Alcohol
Joseph L. Galiber

America was conceived as, and has remained, the noble experiment, the shining bastion of liberties and freedoms for all the world to emulate. Now, in the era when other nations are indeed emulating Americans' craving for freedom, rising from chains and oppression to shake their fists at ancient monoliths, out of frustration

American officials have begun to espouse rank violations of our civil liberties and freedoms.

I realize, of course, that those well-meaning officials say that they are raising their voices for such drastic measures to combat a most pervasive disease, worse than cancer, worse than AIDS: the proliferation of drug use.

But those officials must see, if they and we ever hope to combat drugs, that their every effort to escalate the war against drugs is, at the same time, a confession that the war is being lost. In light of what must inevitably occur, their incursions into civil liberties are as dangerous to our very foundations as they are important to combating the problem.

What we must inevitably do is to eliminate drug trafficking by legalizing narcotics. I realize that some who hear my words think such an idea preposterous, inconceivably simplistic, and naive—a monstrous immorality. Yet each and every device, plan, expenditure, and interdiction thrown into our breastworks fails to stem the tide of drugs. I suggest that legalization—the proper channeling of the deluge, the treatment and calming of the waters—is not only the sole solution, it is inevitable. And so it should be!

When, in the name of fighting the war against drugs, responsible officials suggest arming our police with more powerful automatic weapons, the better to escalate the warfare in our streets; when officials suggest interdicting and shooting out of the sky suspicious planes; when presidential candidates call for doubling the monumental numbers and costs of drug agents; when plans are made for martial law in the capital of our Republic; when the drumbeat for death penalties for drug traffickers is being pounded by otherwise sane and sober leaders; when all of these measures are being espoused despite the fact that we are losing that war, that we are falling back further each day—then I say you must sit back now, right now, and let this message flow over you.

It won't hurt, you can cling tenaciously to your outmoded concept of fighting the losing war, but at least harken to reality.

There is a very simple reason that every person engaged in the front lines of the war has reported that the war is being lost. Millions of our citizens are using drugs every day, right this very minute. All over this country, private citizens are using drugs, buying drugs, craving drugs.

No one can seriously suggest that all the drugs that are smuggled into this country are being stored somewhere in a vast underground cavern, unwanted, unused. Hardly! They are being used. Some estimates put the percentage of citizens over the age of 21 who have at least experimented with drugs at over 40 percent. The drugs are being used by citizens of the United States of America.

Did one of our presidential candidates say that our nation, with one-fifth of the world's population, uses 50 percent of the cocaine in the world? Did another of our presidential candidates suggest the road to solution is a change in values, education? Yes indeed, treatment, rehabilitation, a diminution of the craving, the need, the desire, the curiosity.

Will shooting suspicious planes out of the sky and flaying and quartering every person who deals drugs make the craving of our citizens for the white dream disappear? You can hope it might. But, realistically, an arrest of a dealer does very little for the experimenter, the user, the addict. And surely, in such a lucrative field, others will step into the breach to supply drugs for vast profit.

What we have are *two* very different and very real problems: drug abuse and drug trafficking. Most people fail or refuse to recognize the independent coexistence of those two problems. Perhaps that is the reason for the downfall of our present efforts to stem the tide of drugs.

It is drug trafficking that causes death in the streets and that we spend money to prevent. We spent money on the Coast Guard, ships, planes, agents, spraying crops in foreign countries, and international intrigues. And that addresses only the trafficking.

If by a simple expedient we could eliminate all drug trafficking, so that our nation might turn its attention to the problems of our citizens, turn our resources and efforts to helping them, would that not indeed be the situation we should devoutly desire?

As you listen, you know these words are true. If by midnight tonight we were to legalize narcotics, give them away, free, to those who need them, desire them, in hospitals, under controlled circumstances, then not a plane, not a boat, not a courier would come into this country, beginning at one minute after midnight.

Why? You know the answer. *The profit is gone.* And so, instantly, without anything further, the most violent of our problems, drug trafficking, would stop.

Of course, that wouldn't eliminate drug abuse. But right now we have horrible problems of drug trafficking and all the violence that goes with it. *And* we have drug abuse! Would we not be better off if we could carefully, thoughtfully throw our every effort into eradicating drug abuse only?

The committee asked what were called "key questions" about what drugs would be legalized, who would be eligible to obtain the drugs that would be dispensed or available, who would manufacture them, grow them.

Think of the narcotics industry alongside the alcohol industry. Alcohol, for all those who refuse to admit it, is our most abused drug and it's available everywhere. If you measure drugs by effect or influence on the mind and body, then tobacco isn't a shabby contender for the prize of most abused substance.

The answers to the key questions of the committee, by analogy with the alcohol industry, become automatic. For example:

Question: What narcotics and drugs would be legalized?

Answer: All!

Question: Who would be allowed to buy those narcotics? Would there be an age limit?

Answer: The same limitations as for purchasing alcohol.

Question: Would we sell drugs to people who just want to experiment and encourage them to pick up the habit?

Answer: We would sell drugs in the same fashion and with the same restrictions as we sell alcohol.

Question: Where would drugs be sold?

Answer: In the same places and under the same controls as alcohol.

Question: Where would we obtain our supply of legal drugs?

Answer: In the same way we obtain alcohol; just as there are manufacturers of alcohol, there would be legitimate manufacturers of drugs.

Question: Would private industry be allowed to participate in the market?

Answer: Of course. The same way it does in the market for alcohol.

Question: If drugs became legal, would we allow pilots, railroad workers, and nuclear plant employees to use them?

Answer: Do we permit them to use alcohol?

Question: If drugs were legalized, how would we back up our argument with our children and youth that drugs are harmful? *Answer:* In the same way we do with alcohol.

Every question can be answered in the same fashion, and it is not a mystery that it can be done. Nor is it a mystery that it *should* be done.

We should treat narcotics addiction. We should spend our money treating citizens, curing them of their disease. But what, indeed, does that have to do with eliminating drug trafficking immediately?

The Volstead Act, which made liquor illegal, created violence, warfare, bloodshed, corruption, illicit dealers and sellers on a scale that was unprecedented—*until now.*

And then liquor was legalized. And I ask you, does anyone know a bootlegger running around the streets supplying illicit contraband? Are people worried about drunks mugging them in the streets or breaking into their apartments to get funds to buy a pint of wine?

We now deal with alcohol abuse as a medical problem. Let us deal with the drug problem in the same way. Let us not repeat the mistakes of the past by continuing to escalate a war that is totally unnecessary.

I guarantee, and in your heart's heart you each know, that if you legalize drugs, trafficking will stop immediately. You would then have only one problem to fight.

Granted, it is a vast problem, but as Robert Kennedy opined, "If the alternatives [are] disorder or injustice, the rational choice is injustice. For when there is disorder, we cannot obtain or maintain justice."

So too here, when the disorder and turmoil of drug trafficking surround us, we have no capacity for—and we are not—dealing with the drug problems of our citizens. We must eliminate trafficking, deal with addiction, and help our citizens, not escalate a war that we are losing and that threatens our liberty, our nation, and our very existence.

Joseph L. Galiber is a Democratic state senator from the Bronx.
This article is based on his testimony before the House Select Committee on Narcotics Abuse and Control, September 30, 1988.

Time to License the Drug Trade

The Independent

President George Bush is right to regard drug abuse as the biggest scourge of American society: in announcing a new $7.86 billion strategy yesterday to rescue the nation from it, he described drugs as "the quicksand to our entire society . . . suffocating individuals, families and institutions." But by simply putting more money into the fight against producers, distributors and users, he has chosen the obvious but wrong path.

All previous attempts along similar lines have been counter-productive: the report on which the Bush strategy is based states that drug sales in the United States are now a $110 billion a year industry, bigger than agriculture (though naturally untaxed); and that at least 14 million Americans use illegal drugs. Since the appearance of crack in 1985, the intensive use of cocaine has doubled. Far from being staunched, the supply of drugs has increased. The main effect of any success in reducing it would be to raise prices, and thus dealers' profits and their incentive to push. To stiffen penalties to users, as the White House plan intends, is simply to increase the level of suffering. Treatment and education programmes, which make a genuine contribution to fighting drug abuse, are not being adequately boosted; and the extra money is to be found by cutting social programmes. Yet the more desperate the mental and physical state of America's poor, the more likely they are to use drugs.

Although President Bush has chosen the popular option of yet another crusade against drug pushers and users, the view is spreading that decriminalisation would be a much better approach. When all non-medical dealings in alcohol were prohibited in the United States in 1919, the results were very similar to today's drug trade. Alcohol of often poisonous quality was brewed illicitly; importers were considered criminals and behaved as such; protection rackets, bribes and gang warfare proliferated. Prohibition was the making of the Mafia and other organised crime in the United States. Now that alcohol is legal, its misuse still directly or indirectly kills or wrecks millions of lives, as does the consumption of nicotine. But no one dies (except in some Muslim countries) simply because they import, deal in or enjoy consuming these noxious substances; and governments derive huge tax revenues from licensing and controlling traffic in them.

A recent analysis by the Cato Institute in Washington concluded that the prohibition of drugs criminalised users, forced them into contact with professional criminals, tempted entrepreneurial young people from impoverished backgrounds into a lucrative criminal life, encouraged gang warfare, resulted in people taking impure mixtures in often dangerously strong doses by dangerous methods, and created heavy policing costs. It is, in short, not drug abuse itself which creates the most havoc, but the crime resulting from its prohibition. It is time for the Bush administration, and other Western governments, to contemplate some form of licensed sale of drugs which would deprive the pushers of their market while obliging registered addicts to take treatment. The key to beating the traffic is to remove its prodigious profitability and to deglamorise drug abuse by a heavy programme of public education.

This article is reprinted, with permission, from the *Independent*, September 7, 1989.

A Worthless Crusade

Rufus King

Drug-law reformers missed a fine opportunity last fall when President Bush and drug czar Bennett launched their Great War on Drugs—and then beat a hasty retreat. That retreat would come rapidly is hardly a surprise. We have been unsuccessfully fighting the "war" that Bush chose to redeclare for seven decades. Now, however, Mr. Bennett has rekindled the controversy, calling his critics morally scandalous intellectuals who propose "pseudo-solutions" and speak with "ignorant sneers." Such attacks are not usually made from strength.

Let me start with some numbers Mr. Bennett doesn't often use. The National Institute on Drug Abuse reports that the official 1988 toll of drug-caused deaths in 27 U.S. cities, the best available measure of the nation's "drug problem," was, for cocaine products,

3,308, for heroin and morphine, 2,480, and, of course, for marijuana, zero. "Emergency-room mentions" for cocaine in the same cities totaled only 62,141. For comparison, smoking killed 390,000 last year and alcohol killed at least 100,000. Alcohol is responsible for more fetal damage than crack and remains *the* major menace on our highways.

The last Reagan drug-war budget was $3.4 billion. President Bush's initial request was nearly $6 billion, which he raised to $7.9 billion in his Sept. 5 speech. His strategy called for roughly these proportions: 75 percent for "interdiction" and enforcement, 15 percent for education and prevention, and 10 percent for treatment.

Could anyone be serious about interdicting drug supplies when the plants that produce drugs grow almost anywhere? More than 50 years ago U.S. Narcotics Commissioner Harry Anslinger told Congress that the armed forces and the FBI together couldn't stop the smuggling of illegal drugs across our enormous land and sea borders, and that is still obviously true. And our efforts to stop the growing of drug crops in other countries are an embarrassing tale.

When President Nixon and Attorney General Mitchell came to Washington in 1969 on their law-and-order platform, they faced a problem: law enforcement on the nation's streets is not a federal responsibility. Despite all their purple rhetoric they couldn't *do* much. So they began pumping up the drug menace. But they found that even there the limelight had to be shared with Congress on the domestic front, so they launched interdiction abroad, which they could coordinate with their exclusive control over U.S. foreign policy. Remember Operation Intercept, which virtually closed the Mexican border for a disastrous three weeks? And the pressure the Nixon administration put on Turkey, a minor producer of opium, which nearly drove Turkey out of NATO?

Get-tough enforcement measures, such as "shock incarceration" for users and talk of the headman's ax for pushers, have all been tried before. The long sentences and mandatory minimums of the 1950s choked the courts, strained and disrupted prisons and drove black-market prices higher, with all the attendant corruption and disrespect for law. The latest assault on personal freedom is compulsory testing for nearly everyone, so we can all be kept "drug free."

Drug education and "prevention" are also old stuff, often nothing but sheltered employment for bureaucrats and freeloaders. Generations of education about the dangers of alcohol (in my grade school they used to show us how whisky could cook an egg) have had little effect. Cigarette use is declining not from preventive warnings on packages but through changes in cultural values in the population.

If treatment means honest counseling by a professional in a white coat for those who seek it, and medical relief when addicts require it, treatment programs can indeed help. But that isn't the focus. "Treatment" has often been a euphemism for imprisonment without the protections of the criminal-law system. Today it's "boot camps."

Like smokers and alcoholics, most users of illegal drugs poison themselves because they *want* to be intoxicated. No human force—apart from drug-free imprisonment—and there aren't many U.S. prisons where inmates can't get drugs—can do them much good until they want help. Many eventually "age out"—simply come to a point where they have had enough. But many more drug users, reportedly up to 40 percent in some places, who *are* ready to quit are turned away by long waiting lists and sent back to the street.

Members of Congress and state lawmakers are still trampling one another to outdo the president in lavish outlays and tough posturing. But three weeks after the president's TV performance (he even used a faked exhibit, remember?), the White House began its retreat. Mr. Bennett's deputies were quoted predicting there would be no "overnight success," that the administration's goals were "only guesses" and that the program was almost like "pin the tail on the donkey." And for pure cynical politics, this from a senior White House official: "We have an out (for failure): this was not under the control of the national government."

We reformers are on a roll. Some of the drug-policy rascals may soon be turned out, unless Mr. Bennett comes up with better arguments. It took the nation only 13 years to recognize that Prohibition had been a disastrous mistake. Isn't it about time, after all these decades of folly and failure, that we open our eyes to the realities of this mistake too? Let's hear it for legalization!

Rufus King is a Washington lawyer and the author of *The Drug Hang-Up: America, Fifty-Year Folly.*

This article is reprinted, with permission, from *Newsweek,* January 1, 1990.

A Political Opiate

Lewis H. Lapham

If President Bush's September address to the nation on the topic of drugs can be taken as an example of either his honesty or his courage, I see no reason why I can't look forward to hearing him declare a war against cripples or one-eyed people or red geraniums. It was a genuinely awful speech, rooted in a lie, directed at an imaginary enemy, sustained by false argument, proposing a policy that already had failed, playing to the galleries of prejudice and fear.

The war on drugs is a political war, waged not by scientists and doctors but by police officers and politicians. Under more fortunate circumstances, the prevalence of drugs in American society—not only cocaine and heroin and marijuana but also alcohol and tobacco and sleeping pills—would be properly addressed as a public-health question. The American Medical Association classifies drug addiction as a disease, not as a crime or a moral defect. Nor is addiction contagious, like measles and the flu.

Given the folly and expense of the war on drugs (comparable to the folly and expense of the war in Vietnam), I expect that the United States eventually will arrive at some method of decriminalizing the use of all drugs. The arguments in favor of decriminalization seem to me irrefutable, as do the lessons of experience taught by the failed attempt at the prohibition of alcohol.

But for the time being, as long as the question remains primarily political, the war on drugs serves the purposes of the more reactionary interests within our society (i.e., the defenders of the imagined innocence of a nonexistent past) and transfers the cost of the war to precisely those individuals whom the promoters of the war say they wish to protect.

To politicians in search of sound opinions and sustained applause, this war presents itself as a gift from heaven. Because the human craving for intoxicants cannot be suppressed—not by priests or jailers or acts of Congress—the politicians can bravely confront an allegorical enemy rather than an enemy that takes the corporeal form of the tobacco industry, say, or the Chinese, or the oil and banking lobbies.

The war against drugs provides them with something to say that offends nobody, requires them to do nothing difficult and allows them to postpone, perhaps indefinitely, the more urgent and specific questions about the state of the nation's schools, housing, employment opportunities for young black men—i.e., the conditions to which drug addiction speaks as a tragic symptom, not a cause.

The war on drugs thus becomes the perfect war for people who would rather not fight a war, a war in which the politicians who stand so fearlessly on the side of the good, the true and the beautiful need do nothing else but strike noble poses as protectors of the people and defenders of the public trust.

Their cynicism is implicit in the arithmetic. President Bush in his September speech asked for $7.9 billion to wage his "assault on every front" of the drug war, but the Pentagon allots $5 billion a year to the B-2 program—i.e., to a single weapon. Expressed as a percentage of the federal budget, the new funds assigned to the war on drugs amount to 0.065 percent. Nor does the government offer to do anything boldly military about the legal drugs, principally alcohol and tobacco, that do far more damage to society than all the marijuana and all the cocaine ever smuggled into Florida and California.

(In 1988, American hospitals counted 3,308 deaths attributed to cocaine, as opposed to 390,000 deaths in some way attributable to the use of tobacco and 100,000 deaths directly related to the excessive use of alcohol.)

The drug war, like all wars, sells papers, and the media, like the politicians, ask for nothing better than a safe and profitable menace. The campaign against drugs involves most of the theatrical devices employed by "Miami Vice"—scenes of crimes in progress (almost always dressed up, for salacious effect, with the cameo appearances of one or two prostitutes), melodramatic villains in the Andes, a vocabulary of high-tech military jargon as reassuring as the acronyms in a Tom Clancy novel, the specter of a crazed lumpenproletariat rising in revolt in the nation's cities.

Like camp followers trudging after an army of crusader knights on its way to Jerusalem, the media have in recent months displayed all the garish colors of the profession. Everybody who was anybody set up a booth and offered his or her tears for sale—not only Geraldo and Maury Povich but also, in much the same garish language, Dan Rather (on "48 Hours"), Ted Koppel (on "Nightline") and Sam Donaldson (on "Primetime Live"). In the six weeks between Aug. 1 and Sept. 13, the three television networks combined with the *New York Times* and the *Washington Post* to produce 347 reports from the frontiers of the apocalypse—crack in the cities, cocaine in the suburbs, customs agents seizing pickup trucks on the Mexican border, smugglers named Julio arriving every hour on the hour at Key West.

Most of the journalists writing the dispatches, like most of the columnists handing down the judgments of conscience, knew as much about crack or heroin or cocaine as they knew about the molecular structure of the moons of Saturn. Their ignorance didn't prevent them from coming to the rescue of their own, and the president's, big story.

On "World News Tonight" a few days after the president delivered his address, Peter Jennings, in a tone of voice that was as certain as it was silly (as well as being characteristic of the rest of the propaganda being broadcast over the other networks), said, "Using it even once can make a person crave cocaine for as long as they [sic] live."

So great was the media's excitement, and so determined their efforts to drum up a paying crowd, that hardly anybody bothered to question the premises of the drug war. Without notable exception, the chorus of the big media tuned its instruments to the high metallic pitch of zero tolerance, scorned any truth that didn't echo their own and pasted the smears of derision on the foreheads of the few people, among them Milton Friedman and William Buckley, who had the temerity to suggest that perhaps the war on drugs was both stupid and lost.

The story of the drug war plays to the prejudices of an audience only too eager to believe the worst that can be said about people whom they would rather not know. Because most of the killing allied with the drug trade takes place in the inner cities, and because most of the people arrested for selling drugs prove to be either black or Hispanic, it becomes relatively easy for white people living in safe neighborhoods to blur the distinction between crime and race.

As conditions in the slums deteriorate, which they inevitably must because the government subtracts money from the juvenile-justice and housing programs to finance its drug war, the slums come to look just the way they are supposed to look in the suburban imagination, confirming the fondest suspicions of the governing and possessing classes, justifying the further uses of force and repression. The people who pay the price for the official portrait turn out to be (wonder of wonders) not the members of the prosperous middle class—not the journalists or the academic theorists, not the politicians and government functionaries living behind hedges in Maryland and Virginia—but the law-abiding residents of the inner cities living in the only neighborhoods that they can afford.

It is in the slums of New York that three people, on average, get killed every day—which, over the course of a year, adds up to a higher casualty rate than pertains in Gaza and the West Bank; it is in the slums that the drug trade recruits children to sell narcotics, which is not the result of indigenous villainy but of the nature of the law; it is in the slums that the drug trade has become the exemplary model of finance capitalism for children aspiring to the success of Donald Trump and Samuel Pierce; and it is in the slums that the police experiment with the practice of apartheid, obliging residents of housing projects to carry identity cards and summarily evicting the residents of apartment houses tainted by the presence of drug dealers.

If the folly of the war on drugs could be understood merely as a lesson in political cynicism, or simply as an example of the aplomb with which the venal media can play upon the sentiments of a mob, maybe I would rest content with a few last jokes about the foolishness of the age. But the war on drugs also serves the interests of the state, which, under the pretext of rescuing people from incalculable peril, claims for itself enormously enhanced powers of repression and control.

An opinion poll conducted during the week following President Bush's September address showed 62 percent of the respondents "willing to give up some freedoms" in order to hold America harmless against the scourge of drugs. The government stands more than willing to take them at their word. The war on drugs becomes a useful surrogate for the obsolescent Cold War, now fading into the realm of warm and nostalgic memory. Under the familiar rubrics of constant terror and ceaseless threat, the government subtracts as much as possible from the sum of the nation's civil liberties and imposes de facto martial law on a citizenry that it chooses to imagine as a dangerous rabble.

128

Anybody who doubts this point has only to read the speeches of William Bennett, the commander-in-chief of the Bush administration's war on drugs. Bennett's voice is the voice of an intolerant scold, narrow and shrill and mean-spirited, the voice of a man afraid of liberty and mistrustful of freedom. He believes that it is the government's duty to impose on people a puritanical code of behavior best exemplified by the discipline in place at an unheated boarding school. He never misses the chance to demand more police, more jails, more judges, more arrests, more punishments, more people serving more millennia of "serious time."

In line with Bennett's zeal for coercion, politicians of both parties demand longer jail sentences and harsher laws as well as the right to invade almost everybody's privacy; to search, without a warrant, almost anybody's automobile or boat; to bend the rules of evidence, hire police spies, and attach, again without a warrant, the wires of electronic surveillance. The more obviously the enforcement of the law fails to accomplish its nominal purpose (i.e., as more drugs become more accessible at cheaper prices), the more reasons the Supreme Court finds to warrant the invasion of privacy. In recent years, the court has granted police increasingly autocratic powers— permission (without probable cause) to stop, detain and question travelers passing through the nation's airports in whom the police can see a resemblance to a drug dealer; permission (again without probable cause) to search barns, stop motorists, inspect bank records and tap phones.

The polls suggest that a majority of the American people accept these measures as right and proper. Of the respondents questioned by an ABC/*Washington Post* poll in September, 55 percent supported mandatory drug testing for all Americans, 82 percent favored enlisting the military in the drug war, 52 percent were willing to have their homes searched, and 83 percent favored reporting suspected drug users to the police, even if the suspects happened to be members of their own family.

The enforcement of more and stricter laws requires additional tiers of expensive government, and of the $7.9 billion that President Bush allotted to the war on drugs in September, the bulk of the money swells the budgets of the 58 federal agencies and 74 congressional committees currently engaged, each with its own agenda and armies to feed, on various fronts of the campaign. Which

129

doesn't mean, of course, that the money will be honestly, or intelligently, spent. As was demonstrated plainly by the Reagan administration, the government has a talent for theft and fraud barely distinguishable from the criminal virtuosity of the drug syndicates.

Notwithstanding its habitual incompetence and greed, the government doesn't lightly relinquish the spoils of power seized under the pretexts of apocalypse. What the government grasps, the government seeks to keep and hold. The militarization of the rhetoric supporting the war on drugs rots the public debate with a corrosive silence. People who become accustomed to the arbitrary intrusions of the police also learn to speak more softly in the presence of political authority, to bow and smile and fill out the printed forms with the cowed obsequiousness of musicians playing waltzes at a Mafia wedding.

And for what? To punish people desperate enough or foolish enough to poison themselves with drugs? To exact vengeance on people afflicted with the sickness of addiction and who, to their grief and shame, can find no other way out of the alleys of their despair?

As a consequence of President Bush's war on drugs, society gains nothing except immediate access to an unlimited fund of resentment and unspecific rage. In return for so poor a victory, and in the interests of the kind of people who would build prisons instead of schools, Bush offers the nation the chance to deny its best principles, to corrupt its magistrates and enrich its most vicious and efficient criminals, to repudiate its civil liberties and repent of the habits of freedom. The deal is shabby. For the sake of a vindictive policeman's dream of a quiet and orderly heaven, the country risks losing its constitutional right to its soul.

Lewis H. Lapham is editor of *Harper's* magazine.
This article is abridged, with permission, from *Harper's*, December 1989.

Insisting on Disaster
Anthony Lewis

William Bennett, the Bush drug czar, thinks the United States made a mistake when it repealed Prohibition in 1933. We would be better off if it were a crime to buy a drink.

That, at least, is the logic of Mr. Bennett's latest statement on drug policy. It was a response, in the *Wall Street Journal*, to an open letter from Milton Friedman calling for the decriminalization of drugs. Anyone who wants to know the level of thought behind the Bush-Bennett drug program ought to read it.

Professor Friedman said that relying on the criminal law to stop drug use—the policy of the last many decades—in fact helped to cause the drug scourge. Illegality created obscene profits, corruption, crime: "A replay of our experience with the prohibition of alcoholic beverages."

"The path you propose," Mr. Friedman wrote, "of more police, more jails, use of the military in foreign countries, harsh penalties for drug users, and a whole panoply of repressive measures can only make a bad situation worse." He added that he was revolted by the idea of "turning the United States into an armed camp," with "an army of enforcers empowered to invade the liberty of citizens on slight evidence."

To all this Mr. Bennett gave the back of his hand. Mr. Friedman's argument was "old and familiar," he said. It failed to consider the likelihood that if drugs could be obtained legally, their use would dramatically increase.

"After the repeal of Prohibition," Mr. Bennett said, "consumption of alcohol soared by 350 percent."

So Mr. Bennett, according to his own logic, must regret repeal. It resulted in an immediate increase in drinking, so it was a bad idea.

But that was not the only result of repeal. It did away with speakeasies and rum-runners, with the whole culture of alcohol crime that had given us Al Capone and a new criminal class in this country.

Of course alcohol abuse remains a serious problem. As Mr. Friedman wrote, "Alcohol and tobacco cause many more deaths in users than do drugs." But we have had some success at dealing with the problem by taxation and regulation. Does anyone think we would have more success by once again criminalizing the use of alcohol?

I do not suppose that Mr. Bennett really wants to bring back Prohibition. He just refuses to open his mind to its compelling lesson. In his reply to Mr. Friedman he passed it off in a phrase, saying the analogy between drug and alcohol prohibition was "misunderstood by legalization advocates."

Admitting to ourselves that the law enforcement model has not worked would be no panacea. Willingness to face that reality would be just the beginning of a difficult but at least a sensible path.

The change in policy would have to be made gradually, experimentally, with different ideas in different states. The risks and benefits of such an approach are thoughtfully explored in the Sept. 1 issue of *Science* magazine by Prof. Ethan Nadelmann of Princeton.

Mr. Bennett did not really argue the issue in his letter to Professor Friedman. He substituted pugilism for argument. Government has to teach right and wrong by the criminal law, he said. Only "the liberal elites" disagree.

Liberal elites? Those who have spoken out lately for decriminalization include not only Milton Friedman but two eminent conservative British voices, the *Economist* and the *Financial Times*. Those conservatives understand that criminalizing drugs creates an enormous economic incentive to distribute them.

The *Economist* returned to the point in its last issue, coming up with a telling quotation from John D. Rockefeller Jr. He pushed for Prohibition. But after seeing it in action in the 1920's he wrote:

"That a vast array of lawbreakers has been recruited and financed on a colossal scale . . .; that respect for all law has been greatly lessened; that crime has increased to an unprecedented degree— all this I have slowly and reluctantly come to believe."

It is time for Bill Bennett to open his mind in the same way. He is a student of James Madison, so he knows how crucial it is for public officials to be open to change. And under the bombast he must realize that decriminalizing drugs cannot be honestly dismissed as an "old" idea. The trouble is precisely that our leaders have been too spineless to consider it—too afraid of being called "weak."

Decriminalization, Professor Nadelmann writes in *Science*, has been "dismissed without any attempt to evaluate it openly and objectively. The past 20 years have demonstrated that a drug policy shaped by rhetoric and fear-mongering can only lead to our current disaster."

Anthony Lewis is a columnist for the *New York Times*.

This article is reprinted, with permission, from the *New York Times*, September 24, 1989.

Lazy Thinking on Drugs

Courtland Milloy

Today's "Drug Update, Part X," is a mind-bender: Why are cocaine and heroin illegal while alcohol and tobacco are legal?

- Because cocaine and heroin are more addictive.
- Because cocaine and heroin cause more violent behavior.
- Because America wants to prevent a cocaine/heroin scourge.

And the answer is: All of the above—and they are all wrong.

Yet, as wrong as they are, the above reasons are generally accepted as to why a distinction should be made between alcohol and tobacco on the one hand and illicit substances on the other. That these reasons stand in the face of contradictory facts is just an indicator of how lazy our minds have become when confronting the drug problem in this country.

This short test was based on insights provided by Ethan A. Nadelmann, an assistant professor of politics and public affairs at Princeton University, in an article in the latest *Foreign Policy* magazine titled "U.S. Drug Policy: A Bad Export."

What this society has done, he says, is to make an essentially arbitrary judgment about which "high" is going to be allowed and which is not. The decision had nothing to do with relative safety of the drugs or morality. It was simply the "preference" of the majority for certain drugs and a certain "prejudice" against others.

Nadelmann makes a case that cocaine and heroin are safer than alcohol and tobacco, citing the fact that in 1985 fewer than 3,500 deaths were caused by the first two drugs while alcohol and tobacco cause nearly a half-million deaths every year.

But to justify legalizing some drugs—even the worst of them—while condemning the others, Nadelmann says it was necessary for us to fool ourselves.

"Many Americans make the fallacious assumption that the government would not criminalize certain [drugs] if they were not in fact dangerous," he writes. "Then they jump to the conclusion that any use of those substances is a form of abuse. The government, in its efforts to discourage people from using illicit drugs, has encouraged and perpetuated these misconceptions not just in its rhetoric but also in its purportedly educational materials."

133

Contradictions in accepting one kind of drug over another also resulted in the freezing of our national resolve to deal with the drug problem, he contends. Condoning drugs known to do the most damage while condemning those about which little is known simply made a mockery of all drug laws.

The result is that at least 30 million people regularly break those laws, he says.

"The most unfortunate victims of the drug prohibition policies have been the law-abiding residents of America's ghetto," Nadelmann writes. Because of current antidrug policies, many black areas have become battlegrounds where it is the "aggressive, gun-toting drug dealers who upset residents far more than the addicts nodding in doorways."

He adds that because of increasingly harsh criminal penalties imposed on adult drug dealers, many pushers have turned to widespread recruitment of juveniles as drug traffickers.

"Where once children started dealing drugs only after they had been using them for a few years, today the sequence is often reversed," he says. "Many children start to use illegal drugs now only after they have worked for older drug dealers for a while."

During a recent interview about his article, which I recommend to those who sponsor drug forums and seminars, Nadelmann pointed out that in most black areas "antidrug laws," which have done nothing to reduce the availability of drugs, also have nothing to do with people not using drugs. People choose not to use.

He suggests that now is the time to examine whether our current antidrug policies are causing the city more harm than good.

Courtland Milloy is a columnist for the *Washington Post*.
This article is reprinted, with permission, from the *Washington Post*, April 7, 1988.

Time to Wage a Peace Offensive
The Oakland Tribune

What is to be done about drugs?

America can go on as it has for another three-quarters of a century, destroying life and liberty in the pursuit of drugs, like the

U.S. Army officer in Vietnam who destroyed a village in order to save it.

It can continue harassing, humiliating and jailing drug users in the name of helping them stay away from evil. It can continue fostering violence and corruption in the name of protecting our society.

Or America can begin fighting drugs through peaceful means, taking the problem away from police and jailers and handing it over to doctors and educators.

Legalizing drug use—with certain restrictions—would eliminate the terrible collateral damage wreaked by the war on drugs. It would respect the right of individuals to make personal choices about what they consume, while still holding them responsible for the harm they cause others. It would free up real money for prevention and treatment programs that currently enjoy more lip service than funding. And it would encourage people with problems to seek help rather than take them underground.

Any new approach to drugs must begin by replacing hype and demagoguery with information and analysis. It must discriminate between the uses and misuses of drugs. And it must substitute compassion for punitive enforcement, tolerance for paternalistic moralizing and consistent principles for hypocritical double standards.

It would begin by dropping the distinction between "good" drugs and "bad" drugs. There are only good and bad uses of drugs.

The effects of any drug depend on dosage, frequency, individual chemistry, mode of administration and social setting. Aspirin can kill pain in small quantities and kill you in larger quantities. The same goes for heroin, although it causes less organic damage than aspirin. Coca has mild medicinal qualities when chewed by Andean peasants and far more potent and dangerous effects when smoked in the form of crack. Pure cocaine is a valuable anesthetic favored by surgeons for its long duration, low toxicity and ability to constrict blood vessels.

It follows that not every use of illicit drugs is necessarily damaging, despite the potential hazards. Millions of Americans, however unwisely, have tried them without harm. To put things in perspective, more people died in 1985 from appendicitis (570) than from cocaine (563). That same year, 337 people aged 24 and under died in swimming pool accidents. No one died of marijuana. All illicit drugs together accounted for 3,562 deaths in 1985. Alcohol, on the other hand, took 100,000 lives and tobacco claimed another 300,000.

Addiction is a problem with some illicit drugs, though medical understanding is far from complete. Some drugs produce physical withdrawal effects; others stimulate psychological craving only. But even heroin, an especially addictive drug, doesn't enslave most casual users. During periods of heroin shortages, long-term users typically switch to other drugs without much trauma.

Of the 250,000 U.S. soldiers in Vietnam who used heroin, more than 90 percent were able to quit without assistance and only 1 percent used heroin again. Although addiction and withdrawal can be unfortunate and painful, they would be far more bearable and treatable without the overlay of crime, deceit and social stigma that laws create today.

Irrational fears and stereotypes, not sound medical evidence, prompted politicians to make unfamiliar drugs illegal and their users into criminals. A federal report warned in 1910 that "cocaine is often the direct incentive of the crime of rape by Negroes in the South and other sections of the country." Southern sheriffs switched to .38-caliber pistols because they heard that cocaine-crazed black criminals were invulnerable to smaller calibers. Opium and heroin were associated with the "yellow peril," marijuana with Mexicans.

Harry Anslinger, head of the Federal Bureau of Narcotics, got Congress to ban the sale of marijuana in 1937 with his tales of "reefer madness." "If the hideous monster Frankenstein came face to face with the monster Marijuana, he would drop dead of fright," Anslinger declared.

The best medical experts of his time had concluded that "moderate use . . . produces no injurious effects on the mind" and that marijuana was not addictive. A military panel in 1925 even approved its use by U.S. soldiers in Panama after examining its effects. The American Medical Association, intrigued by its possible medical benefits, strongly opposed banning marijuana. But Congress acted on the devil theory instead.

Legalizing drugs wouldn't be a panacea. Many people would continue to use them recklessly and suffer the consequences. Some misguided newcomers would surely join their ranks. But scare scenarios of a prostrate, addicted nation have no basis.

For one thing, drugs are already available to almost anyone who wants them. Eighty-eight percent of high school seniors say they can easily lay their hands on marijuana; 71 percent say the same for amphetamines. Nearly half can get cocaine without trouble and more than a fifth say heroin is no problem either. Three-fifths of seniors have tried illicit drugs at least once. As Rep. Charles Rangel, D-N.Y., and head of the House Select Committee on Narcotics Abuse and Control, said, "They are selling cocaine on the streets of New York like you sell candy to a baby."

Even so, the good news is that drug use seems to be falling. The number of 18- to 25-year-olds who used cocaine in any given month fell from 9.3 percent in 1979 to 7.6 percent in 1985, the last year for which data are available. Marijuana use plummeted from 35.4 percent to 21.6 percent. Cocaine use among high school seniors dropped by a third from 1986 to 1987. Cigarette smoking, though both legal and addictive, is falling fast in the general population. These data suggest that social attitudes and the cultural climate influence drug use more than laws.

Where drugs are legal, they don't spread like the plague. The Netherlands legalized marijuana in 1978. Use among 13- to 25-year-olds fell from 15 percent in 1976 to 2 percent in 1983. Legalization took away its allure. "Because society hasn't defined it as a problem, it isn't a problem," observed Peter Cohen, a psychologist who advises the Dutch government. Alaska legalized personal use of marijuana by court order in the mid-1970s without suffering ill effects.

As for cocaine and heroin, the effects of legalization can best be gauged by America's own experience. Before 1915, both were legal. Cocaine was highly popular in the 1880s, but fell out of favor as people learned of its drawbacks. By 1900, some 250,000 addicts used heroin; the number fell slowly thereafter even while the drug remained legal. Today America has about as many addicts relative to the total population.

A compassionate approach to drugs would give all users access to treatment-on-demand without making them wait for months for help as they often do today. Such an approach would fund treatment, education and research programs by taxing drug sales so society, not criminals, could profit. It would try to cope with the psychological and medical issues facing problem drug users rather than compounding their misery with legal sanctions.

137

Laws would continue to bar sales to minors and would limit distribution, say, to pharmacy counters to prevent impulse buying at vending machines or supermarkets. They would ensure proper regulation of drug purity. They would ban advertising to limit demand. (Indeed, with pushers priced out of business, no one would have financial motives to tout drugs anymore.) They would impose tough sanctions for driving or engaging in other dangerous activities while under the influence of drugs.

Above all, America would not endorse or minimize the risks of taking drugs, any more than it now endorses Nazis or Communists by tolerating their political activities. On the contrary, our society must always champion the ability of human beings to realize their full potential best when their free will and reasoning faculties are unimpaired by drugs. But it cannot teach that lesson convincingly so long as it tries to deny free will through unreasoning drug laws.

This article is reprinted, with permission, from the *Oakland Tribune*, June 24, 1988.

To Fight the Crime and Corruption Surrounding Drugs, Legalize Them

Ned Pattison

For the last two years, the American public has been bombarded with the issue of illegal drugs. Every major newsweekly, every TV network, and every local newspaper has featured frequent stories on the problem of cocaine and crack.

Politicians, eager for a no-lose issue, especially one that pushes other, more difficult issues off the political agenda, have waded right in. Candidates across the nation vie for the position of being tougher on drugs than their opponents, sometimes by challenging them to submit to urine tests. Each has his own proposal to pursue the "war" on drugs.

Congress, unable to deal with the budget and other pressing issues, will enact, almost unanimously, a drug bill calling for massive expenditures of money, involvement of the U.S. Armed Forces, and the erosion of many fundamental civil liberties. Woe to the representatives with the courage to vote no. The whole country has somehow become engaged in an anti-drug frenzy.

The solution, if any, involves changing the culture, and that means that it is by nature, a long-term one, with no quick legislative or political fix. Unfortunately, in American politics, the surest road to defeat is for a candidate to suggest that some problem has no legislative solution. It is always the better part of political wisdom to at least "try something."

Drug abuse is not a new problem, and the political response is always the same. Tougher laws, more police, harsher penalties. Those "solutions" have not only not worked to reduce drug abuse, but have had the result of creating other problems that are in many ways far worse. Organized crime has prospered on drugs; corruption of public officials has blossomed; street crime has vastly increased; expenditures for the criminal justice system have sky-rocketed, without appreciable impact on drug use.

None of this should be a surprise. All you have to do is go back to the 1920s for a similar experience. In those days, the country decided that alcohol was a terrible problem. And it was! So we amended the U.S. Constitution to prohibit alcohol. Then we poured the energies of the FBI and the local police into the effort. The result? Alcohol abuse continued to be a problem, Americans lost their respect for law, organized crime flourished as never before, and corruption of public officials soared. Finally, after about a dozen years of the "noble experiment," we repealed the amendment. The problems caused by alcohol abuse got no better—nor any worse. Alcohol-related crime and expenditures to combat it decreased, and organized crime had to look for more fertile fields.

The drug problem has no "solution," any more than the alcohol problem, or for that matter, the pornography, prostitution, or gambling problems. All share one characteristic. Both the buyers and the sellers engage in the activity voluntarily. In the case of most crimes, one of the parties is the victim, and after the crime is committed, the victim makes a complaint to the police. Not so with so-called "victimless crimes." It is difficult enough to catch and punish the perpetrator of a crime with a victim. But the difficulties in catching and punishing criminals where no one involved in the crime makes a complaint are orders of magnitude greater.

Since such activity is voluntary, prohibiting it only serves to increase the price without raising the basic cost of the product. This ensures enormous profits for those willing to violate the law. And those profits will inevitably lead to corruption so long as human beings are human.

What would happen if we decided, as in the case of alcohol, to surrender, to repeal the laws outlawing drugs?

Once selling drugs was no longer illegal, as in the case of other goods, competition would drastically lower the price. With no possibility of enormous profits, organized crime would no longer be interested. With no need to bribe public officials, corruption, at least from this source, would disappear.

With the price greatly reduced, what would be the effect on drug usage? Once again, look at the experience of the "noble experiment." After repeal, the price of alcohol, even with a very stiff tax, went way down. Alcohol use increased, but alcohol abuse remained about the same.

Obviously, a problem as serious as the drug problem can't just be ignored. But the intuitive solution of prohibition has been proven to cause problems worse than the problem we set out to solve without solving the problem itself.

The reality is that large parts of the crime problem, the corruption problem, and the AIDS problem wouldn't exist if it weren't for the fact that drugs are illegal and thus extremely profitable. The same is true of the current problems with Colombia, Peru, Panama, and Bolivia. Budgetary problems, at the national, state, and local levels would be lessened.

Legalization of drugs offers no solution to the drug problem. But it does offer a significant lessening of four other problems. The choice between having one problem or five problems is obvious.

Certainly we should be willing to increase society's efforts in the area of prevention by education, and where that fails, rehabilitation and treatment. The solution to a cultural problem is to change the culture; and changing the culture is not something that can be done overnight.

Certainly legalization would not include children, any more than was the case for alcohol. Prevention of drug abuse by children will continue to require a certain amount of law enforcement activity. That should be a whole lot easier when the enormous profit is taken out of the business.

140

In a free society, if an adult decides that he wants to get drunk, or blow his nose off his face with cocaine, so long as he doesn't do it while he is driving his car or performing surgery, that's his choice. On one level, I can feel sympathy for a Len Bias who destroys a life with great potential. On another level, I really can't get too upset. He, or others who have and will intentionally do damage to themselves, will simply have to accept the consequences of their own behavior.

Ned Pattison is a lawyer in Troy, New York, and served in Congress from 1975 to 1979.

This article is reprinted, with permission, from the *Schenectady Gazette*, September 23, 1989.

A Battlefield View of War on Drugs

Mike Royko

John is a white Chicago cop. He doesn't want his full name used because what he has to say might not please his superiors, although many probably agree with him.

"I'm a sergeant and I've worked on the West Side by choice most of my career. So I know something about the problem of drugs. I think I know more about it than some of the people who do a lot of talking about winning the drug war and make the laws and set our national policies, but have never been on the street where everything is happening.

"For years I've been advocating, mostly to my friends, the legalization of drugs and using the billions we'd save from trying to fight the import and sales, to cure those who want to be cured.

"The way things go now, the courts will sentence drug offenders and people who steal to get drug money to rehabilitation as a condition of probation.

"But what happens when they want to go straight and can't get into a program for six months, which is very common? I'll tell you what. They go right back to their friends and habits. So instead of spending all those billions pretending you're doing something, some of the money could be used for rehab, some of it for ad campaigns not to use it, the way it's done with cigarettes and liquor.

"We'd still have laws against the sale to minors. You know, it pains me to see how rich drug laws have made punks and white collar opportunists. But once the profits aren't there, the punks and the others are out of business.

"On the West Side, kids used to complain that we stopped them because they were black and driving a new Cadillac. That was true. Most often the car was stolen and we had to chase them.

"But now that's changed. Now the cars belong to them and they've paid cash. And some of them aren't even old enough to drive.

"Those of us in law enforcement look like fools trying to fight a battle we can't win. And that just breeds contempt for law and order.

"You know, even if we were able to stop the coke from Colombia and Peru, it wouldn't change things. It would come in from somewhere else. And if we stopped that, it still wouldn't change because now they can make this synthetic stuff right here. They're doing it already.

"The problem is the demand. And the only thing for sure is that where there is a demand, it will be satisfied. That's a basic market principle, and that's why all the arguments against legalizing and controlling drugs are nonsense.

"I'll tell you what the biggest change in the last four or five years has been. It's the drug dealers themselves.

"Now we have 13-year-old dealers who make more than me. They go out and sell, then they give some of the money to mom, who maybe lives in the [Chicago Housing Authority] or some dump. She needs it to make ends meet.

"How can President Bush fault someone who lives in a drafty apartment and is wanting for food and has no chance for a decent education or a job for selling drugs?

"How are you going to convince the kids to get back to school so they can be a factory worker, or get a low paying job in a fast food place, or be unemployed, when they can sell drugs for big money?

"Then they're going to have kids and they won't be able to steer them away from drugs or get them to go to school because they can't lead by example. If you're going to have values and morals, they have to come by example. And that's why we have all the casual violence out there, the disregard for life and death.

"The way we're going at this thing reminds me of Vietnam. A quagmire. Lives lost, then we pack up and leave.

"One of the reasons we study history is to learn from our own mistakes. Well, it looks like we didn't learn anything from Prohibition.

"I keep reading that every poll shows that most people are against any kind of legalizing of drugs.

"You know what that tells me? It tells me that most people who get polled don't know what the hell is going on out here."

That's one cop's opinion. But I suspect it is also the opinion of thousands of other cops in Chicago, New York, L.A., and in most cities where the problems are the same.

Since they're the ones who are actually fighting this no-win war, I respect their opinions more than the word-warriors in Washington who have never been closer to Chicago's West Side, or New York's Bronx, or L.A.'s Watts than their TV sets can get them.

Mike Royko is a nationally syndicated columnist.

This article is reprinted, with permission, from the *Chicago Tribune*, September 15, 1989.

Decriminalize Drugs

Thomas Sowell

When a stampede gets under way, some people want to join it. Others want to see where it is headed. The latest stampede is "the war on drugs" launched by President Bush.

The president has used the language of the stampede—be "angry," be "united," be "determined" and "get involved." He has called drugs "the toughest domestic challenge we've faced in decades."

Before we get caught up in this stampede, we need to do something the president did not ask us to do—stop and think. What does the drug problem consist of and how will the federal government's new crusade make things better?

There are some very different things lumped together as "the drug problem." There is the harm done directly to those who become drug addicts. There is the harm done to innocent victims. And there is the harm done to the basic fabric of American life. Which of these things will be helped—and which will be hurt—by the so-called "war on drugs"?

President Bush says that there are about a million regular users of crack. That is a lot of people and a lot of devastation of mind and body. Most of those people choose to be crack users and many will continue to choose to live that kind of life—short and sordid as it may be.

There is no point kidding ourselves that these hard-core crack addicts got that way because they just didn't know any better. Drug "education" programs are not likely to save them. This is only one of the ways the so-called "war on drugs" proceeds as if it is OK to impose open-ended costs on the vast majority of Americans who are not cocaine addicts, in hopes of doing something for that fraction of one percent who are.

In addition to the hard-core cocaine addicts, there are seven million "casual users." But this number is going down. Why is a declining number of cocaine users "the toughest domestic challenge we've faced in decades"?

Let's turn to the truly innocent victims of drugs. Those on the front line are the people in whose neighborhoods the real drug wars are fought between rival gangs. These drug-dealing hoodlums are often armed to the teeth and ready to spray the area with bullets at any time, regardless of whether there are children on the streets. The innocent victims also include those who try to enforce drug laws in Third World countries where much of the drug traffic originates.

Unlike drug deaths among addicts, these deaths are not due to the drugs themselves but to laws that make drugs illegal and prescribe heavy penalties. The war on drugs approach simply raises the stakes still further. This raises both the price of drugs and the dangers of getting caught—and thus virtually guarantees

144

more desperate fighting and more innocent people caught in the crossfire.

Even those living far from the neighborhoods that become drug battlegrounds are victims, as the basic fabric of American life is threatened. Crime and corruption spread far and wide when drugs are criminalized, just as a ban on alcohol corrupted law enforcement agencies, the courts and politicians during the Prohibition era. Whatever else the late J. Edgar Hoover was, he was a shrewd man—and he resisted all efforts to get his FBI involved in drug-law enforcement.

Mr. Bush's "coordinated, cooperative commitment of all federal agencies" in the war on drugs ignores the danger that all these agencies—including the military—will become targets of corruption and infiltration by the international drug cartels. They already are in places like Colombia.

Some parts of the president's plan—more prisons, more courts, more prosecutors—make sense. What would make still more sense would be to admit that we are not God, that we cannot live other people's lives or save people who don't want to be saved, and to take the profits out of drugs by decriminalizing them. That is what destroyed the bootleggers' gangs after Prohibition was repealed.

Thomas Sowell is a senior research fellow at the Hoover Institution.

This article is reprinted, with permission, from the *San Francisco Examiner*, September 18, 1989.

Stop the War on Drugs—Legalize Them

Arnold S. Trebach

There's a historic opening in the public consciousness: For the first time, people are willing to consider legalization as a way to end the drug wars. George Bush and Michael Dukakis have a chance to make history during the next year and a half if only they are able to summon the courage and gather the insight into how to push forward with these ideas. Such innovation would be the equivalent of Richard Nixon's surprise triumph in making peace with Red China, perhaps his greatest accomplishment.

Of course, the subject of legalization must be treated very delicately during this campaign by the presidential candidates and by other office seekers. Few politicians should risk coming out flatly for legalization lest they be accused by their opponents of being in league with the drug pushers. At the same time, all of them should be able to resist the urge to out-Rambo each other, an urge to which Bush now seems to be succumbing.

They should tone down the negative drug-war hysteria in their speeches and emphasize such positive programs as education and treatment, on which the Reagan administration has penny-pinched. And all thoughful candidates should welcome the dialogue on reforming current drug policies being promoted by such gutsy politicians as Baltimore Mayor Kurt L. Schmoke and Rep. Fortney H. "Pete" Stark, D-Calif.

Confidential plans can be made now by candidates that will set out peaceful models of drug-policy reform as the basis for a series of experiments after the election.

Legalization does not mean that we must drop all the drug laws at once. As I use it, the term encompasses any approach that reduces the role of criminal law and of extremist ideology, such as that which labels drug users as accomplices to murder. One starting step would be for the next president to order that drug laws be selectively enforced, as are the nation's sex laws.

Currently, there are statutes criminalizing many sexual acts that are eagerly and regularly committed privately by millions of consenting adults, including members of Congress, judges, police, prosecutors and prison guards. Our compromise has been to leave the sex laws on the books—public hypocrisy being much desired in matters of morals and pleasure—but to enforce these laws only against the most harmful illegal acts, such as child molestation and rape.

How would this work for drugs? We can look to the Netherlands for the answer. Despite whatever you may have heard, all of the drugs illegal in America are illegal in Holland, including marijuana. Unlike the U.S., the Dutch government rejects the very idea of a war on drugs, viewing it as destructive. As Dr. C. F. Ruter, a criminal law professor at the University of Amsterdam, said

146

recently at a Drug Policy Forum on Capitol Hill: "These users and addicts are part of our Dutch family."

Starting from this humane viewpoint, Dutch criminal justice officials and lawyers have developed an extensive set of prosecutorial guidelines that are the heart of their system. Marijuana and hashish are treated as if they were fully legal when they appear to be possessed for personal use or small sales. Dealers who sell in large quantities, or who engage in violence or organized crime, are prosecuted.

Similarly, possession of a small amount of hard drugs is ignored. Addicts are approached by the Dutch government as decent citizens who need health care. Unions of addicts, or "junkie bonds," function throughout the country as a legitimate interest group. The junkie bonds operate clean needle and advice programs for addicts. Some doctors provide methadone and morphine to them.

And the results? Impressive. While there is some crime by addicts and dealers, it is moderate by American standards. So also is the rate of hard drug use. Marijuana use is even lower on a comparative basis. Dutch youth seem bored with the readily available pot and use it at a rate less than 10 percent that of American young people.

But perhaps the most important benefit from the Dutch model is how a straightforward approach to drugs has kept the rate of AIDS among addicts very low. In Holland, the number of intravenous drug users with the disease is tiny compared to the U.S. and many other countries.

Professor Ruter's advice at the Capitol Hill forum: Pull the criminal law and the police "back into the corner." He doesn't suggest legalizing any drugs, but calls for a waiting period to see how effective a more humanitarian approach turns out to be. If the new system does not work, law enforcement can resume and no laws have to be changed. If the new system works, real changes in the law should be made.

But I would propose some first steps toward legalization. Congress could pass a law directing that heroin, marijuana and other feared drugs be made available to millions of Americans when their doctors prescribe them as medicines. England provides the best model of the extensive use of heroin as an effective pain killer in the treatment of some patients, including those with terminal cancer. Such a measure would help innocent sick people who have nothing to do with the drug scene. To its everlasting shame, the Reagan administration has generally opposed such compassionate reforms.

But we don't have to look abroad for examples of reasonable reform. In 1975, the Alaskan Supreme Court interpreted the right of privacy in the state constitution to allow adults to grow and possess marijuana for personal use in the privacy of the home. Within these constraints, the drug is legal, not simply decriminalized as it is in 10 other states.

The Alaskan approach has worked well and has not caused any measurable harm to the people of that state, especially its children. Subsequently, the Alaska legislature has rejected several attempts to recriminalize marijuana.

Also sitting under our noses is the alcohol repeal model of 1933. The constitutional amendment that repealed alcohol prohibition did not make alcohol legal. Rather, it allowed each state to choose the model of alcohol control that best suited the needs of its citizenry. While this is the most radical of any idea here proposed, it rests on a conservative American principle: states' rights.

Alcohol remains a difficult problem, especially in terms of public health, but the crime, corruption and violence associated with prohibition of this toxic, yet legal, drug have virtually disappeared.

Even though it may be politically impossible in the near future, our next president and his congressional allies should consider a law that would allow the states to experiment with new forms of drug control. It is difficult to conjure up a situation in which any state government could do worse than what the federal government is doing now. Indeed, the implementation of any of these ideas, alone or in combination, should greatly improve a worsening drug situation.

Arnold S. Trebach is president of the Drug Policy Foundation.
This article is reprinted, with permission, from the *Los Angeles Herald Examiner*, June 26, 1988.

About the Editor

David Boaz is executive vice president of the Cato Institute. He previously served as editor of *New Guard* magazine and executive director of the Council for a Competitive Economy. He writes frequently for such publications as the *New York Times*, the *Washington Post*, the *Wall Street Journal*, and the *Chicago Tribune*. He is the editor of *Left, Right, and Babyboom: America's New Politics* and *Assessing the Reagan Years* and coeditor with Edward H. Crane of *An American Vision: Policies for the '90s*.

Cato Institute

Founded in 1977, the Cato Institute is a public policy research foundation dedicated to broadening the parameters of policy debate to allow consideration of more options that are consistent with the traditional American principles of limited government, individual liberty, and peace. Toward that goal, the Institute strives to achieve greater involvement of the intelligent, concerned lay public in questions of policy and the proper role of government.

The Institute is named for *Cato's Letters*, pamphlets that were widely read in the American Colonies in the early 18th century and played a major role in laying the philosophical foundation for the revolution that followed. Since that revolution, civil and economic liberties have been eroded as the number and complexity of social problems have grown.

To counter this trend the Cato Institute undertakes an extensive publications program dealing with the complete spectrum of policy issues. Books, monographs, and shorter studies are commissioned to examine the federal budget, Social Security, regulation, NATO, international trade, and a myriad of other issues. Major policy conferences are held throughout the year, from which papers are published thrice yearly in the *Cato Journal*.

In order to maintain an independent posture, the Cato Institute accepts no government funding. Contributions are received from foundations, corporations, and individuals, and other revenue is generated from the sale of publications. The Institute is a nonprofit, tax-exempt, educational foundation under Section 501(c)3 of the Internal Revenue Code.

CATO INSTITUTE
224 Second St., S.E.
Washington, D.C. 20003